FREE Study Skills Videos/DVD Offer

Dear Customer,

Thank you for your purchase from Mometrix! We consider it an honor and a privilege that you have purchased our product and we want to ensure your satisfaction.

As part of our ongoing effort to meet the needs of test takers, we have developed a set of Study Skills Videos that we would like to give you for FREE. These videos cover our *best practices* for getting ready for your exam, from how to use our study materials to how to best prepare for the day of the test.

All that we ask is that you email us with feedback that would describe your experience so far with our product. Good, bad, or indifferent, we want to know what you think!

To get your FREE Study Skills Videos, you can use the **QR code** below, or send us an **email** at studyvideos@mometrix.com with *FREE VIDEOS* in the subject line and the following information in the body of the email:

- The name of the product you purchased.
- Your product rating on a scale of 1-5, with 5 being the highest rating.
- Your feedback. It can be long, short, or anything in between. We just want to know your impressions and experience so far with our product. (Good feedback might include how our study material met your needs and ways we might be able to make it even better. You could highlight features that you found helpful or features that you think we should add.)

If you have any questions or concerns, please don't hesitate to contact me directly.

Thanks again!

Sincerely,

Jay Willis
Vice President
jay.willis@mometrix.com
1-800-673-8175

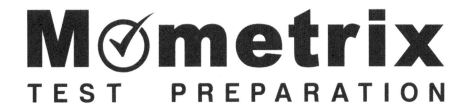

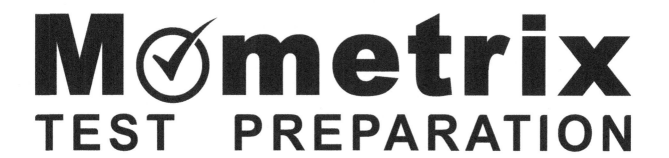

MBLEx

Test Prep 2025-2026

3 Full-Length Practice Exams

Secrets Study Guide for the FSMTB Massage and Bodywork License with Detailed Answer Explanations

8th Edition

Written and edited by Matthew Bowling

Printed in the United States of America

This paper meets the requirements of ANSI/NISO Z39.48-1992 (Permanence of Paper).

Mometrix offers volume discount pricing to institutions. For more information or a price quote, please contact our sales department at sales@mometrix.com or 888-248-1219.

Mometrix Media LLC is not affiliated with or endorsed by any official testing organization. All organizational and test names are trademarks of their respective owners.

ISBN 13: 978-1-5167-2773-5
ISBN 10: 1-5167-2773-8

DEAR FUTURE EXAM SUCCESS STORY

First of all, **THANK YOU** for purchasing Mometrix study materials!

Second, congratulations! You are one of the few determined test-takers who are committed to doing whatever it takes to excel on your exam. **You have come to the right place.** We developed these study materials with one goal in mind: to deliver you the information you need in a format that's concise and easy to use.

In addition to optimizing your guide for the content of the test, we've outlined our recommended steps for breaking down the preparation process into small, attainable goals so you can make sure you stay on track.

We've also analyzed the entire test-taking process, identifying the most common pitfalls and showing how you can overcome them and be ready for any curveball the test throws you.

Standardized testing is one of the biggest obstacles on your road to success, which only increases the importance of doing well in the high-pressure, high-stakes environment of test day. Your results on this test could have a significant impact on your future, and this guide provides the information and practical advice to help you achieve your full potential on test day.

Your success is our success

We would love to hear from you! If you would like to share the story of your exam success or if you have any questions or comments in regard to our products, please contact us at **800-673-8175** or **support@mometrix.com**.

Thanks again for your business and we wish you continued success!

Sincerely,
The Mometrix Test Preparation Team

Need more help? Check out our flashcards at:
http://mometrixflashcards.com/MBLEx

TABLE OF CONTENTS

Introduction

Thank you for purchasing this resource! You have made the choice to prepare yourself for a test that could have a huge impact on your future, and this guide is designed to help you be fully ready for test day. Obviously, it's important to have a solid understanding of the test material, but you also need to be prepared for the unique environment and stressors of the test, so that you can perform to the best of your abilities.

For this purpose, the first section that appears in this guide is the **Secret Keys**. We've devoted countless hours to meticulously researching what works and what doesn't, and we've boiled down our findings to the five most impactful steps you can take to improve your performance on the test. We start at the beginning with study planning and move through the preparation process, all the way to the testing strategies that will help you get the most out of what you know when you're finally sitting in front of the test.

We recommend that you start preparing for your test as far in advance as possible. However, if you've bought this guide as a last-minute study resource and only have a few days before your test, we recommend that you skip over the first two Secret Keys since they address a long-term study plan.

If you struggle with **test anxiety**, we strongly encourage you to check out our recommendations for how you can overcome it. Test anxiety is a formidable foe, but it can be beaten, and we want to make sure you have the tools you need to defeat it.

Secret Key #1 – Plan Big, Study Small

There's a lot riding on your performance. If you want to ace this test, you're going to need to keep your skills sharp and the material fresh in your mind. You need a plan that lets you review everything you need to know while still fitting in your schedule. We'll break this strategy down into three categories.

Information Organization

Start with the information you already have: the official test outline. From this, you can make a complete list of all the concepts you need to cover before the test. Organize these concepts into groups that can be studied together, and create a list of any related vocabulary you need to learn so you can brush up on any difficult terms. You'll want to keep this vocabulary list handy once you actually start studying since you may need to add to it along the way.

Time Management

Once you have your set of study concepts, decide how to spread them out over the time you have left before the test. Break your study plan into small, clear goals so you have a manageable task for each day and know exactly what you're doing. Then just focus on one small step at a time. When you manage your time this way, you don't need to spend hours at a time studying. Studying a small block of content for a short period each day helps you retain information better and avoid stressing over how much you have left to do. You can relax knowing that you have a plan to cover everything in time. In order for this strategy to be effective though, you have to start studying early and stick to your schedule. Avoid the exhaustion and futility that comes from last-minute cramming!

Study Environment

The environment you study in has a big impact on your learning. Studying in a coffee shop, while probably more enjoyable, is not likely to be as fruitful as studying in a quiet room. It's important to keep distractions to a minimum. You're only planning to study for a short block of time, so make the most of it. Don't pause to check your phone or get up to find a snack. It's also important to **avoid multitasking**. Research has consistently shown that multitasking will make your studying dramatically less effective. Your study area should also be comfortable and well-lit so you don't have the distraction of straining your eyes or sitting on an uncomfortable chair.

 The time of day you study is also important. You want to be rested and alert. Don't wait until just before bedtime. Study when you'll be most likely to comprehend and remember. Even better, if you know what time of day your test will be, set that time aside for study. That way your brain will be used to working on that subject at that specific time and you'll have a better chance of recalling information.

Finally, it can be helpful to team up with others who are studying for the same test. Your actual studying should be done in as isolated an environment as possible, but the work of organizing the information and setting up the study plan can be divided up. In between study sessions, you can discuss with your teammates the concepts that you're all studying and quiz each other on the details. Just be sure that your teammates are as serious about the test as you are. If you find that your study time is being replaced with social time, you might need to find a new team.

Secret Key #2 – Make Your Studying Count

You're devoting a lot of time and effort to preparing for this test, so you want to be absolutely certain it will pay off. This means doing more than just reading the content and hoping you can remember it on test day. It's important to make every minute of study count. There are two main areas you can focus on to make your studying count.

Retention

It doesn't matter how much time you study if you can't remember the material. You need to make sure you are retaining the concepts. To check your retention of the information you're learning, try recalling it at later times with minimal prompting. Try carrying around flashcards and glance at one or two from time to time or ask a friend who's also studying for the test to quiz you.

To enhance your retention, look for ways to put the information into practice so that you can apply it rather than simply recalling it. If you're using the information in practical ways, it will be much easier to remember. Similarly, it helps to solidify a concept in your mind if you're not only reading it to yourself but also explaining it to someone else. Ask a friend to let you teach them about a concept you're a little shaky on (or speak aloud to an imaginary audience if necessary). As you try to summarize, define, give examples, and answer your friend's questions, you'll understand the concepts better and they will stay with you longer. Finally, step back for a big picture view and ask yourself how each piece of information fits with the whole subject. When you link the different concepts together and see them working together as a whole, it's easier to remember the individual components.

Finally, practice showing your work on any multi-step problems, even if you're just studying. Writing out each step you take to solve a problem will help solidify the process in your mind, and you'll be more likely to remember it during the test.

Modality

Modality simply refers to the means or method by which you study. Choosing a study modality that fits your own individual learning style is crucial. No two people learn best in exactly the same way, so it's important to know your strengths and use them to your advantage.

For example, if you learn best by visualization, focus on visualizing a concept in your mind and draw an image or a diagram. Try color-coding your notes, illustrating them, or creating symbols that will trigger your mind to recall a learned concept. If you learn best by hearing or discussing information, find a study partner who learns the same way or read aloud to yourself. Think about how to put the information in your own words. Imagine that you are giving a lecture on the topic and record yourself so you can listen to it later.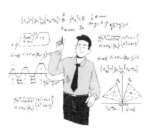

For any learning style, flashcards can be helpful. Organize the information so you can take advantage of spare moments to review. Underline key words or phrases. Use different colors for different categories. Mnemonic devices (such as creating a short list in which every item starts with the same letter) can also help with retention. Find what works best for you and use it to store the information in your mind most effectively and easily.

3

Secret Key #3 – Practice the Right Way

Your success on test day depends not only on how many hours you put into preparing, but also on whether you prepared the right way. It's good to check along the way to see if your studying is paying off. One of the most effective ways to do this is by taking practice tests to evaluate your progress. Practice tests are useful because they show exactly where you need to improve. Every time you take a practice test, pay special attention to these three groups of questions:

- The questions you got wrong
- The questions you had to guess on, even if you guessed right
- The questions you found difficult or slow to work through

This will show you exactly what your weak areas are, and where you need to devote more study time. Ask yourself why each of these questions gave you trouble. Was it because you didn't understand the material? Was it because you didn't remember the vocabulary? Do you need more repetitions on this type of question to build speed and confidence? Dig into those questions and figure out how you can strengthen your weak areas as you go back to review the material.

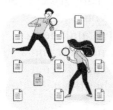 Additionally, many practice tests have a section explaining the answer choices. It can be tempting to read the explanation and think that you now have a good understanding of the concept. However, an explanation likely only covers part of the question's broader context. Even if the explanation makes perfect sense, **go back and investigate** every concept related to the question until you're positive you have a thorough understanding.

As you go along, keep in mind that the practice test is just that: practice. Memorizing these questions and answers will not be very helpful on the actual test because it is unlikely to have any of the same exact questions. If you only know the right answers to the sample questions, you won't be prepared for the real thing. **Study the concepts** until you understand them fully, and then you'll be able to answer any question that shows up on the test.

It's important to wait on the practice tests until you're ready. If you take a test on your first day of study, you may be overwhelmed by the amount of material covered and how much you need to learn. Work up to it gradually.

On test day, you'll need to be prepared for answering questions, managing your time, and using the test-taking strategies you've learned. It's a lot to balance, like a mental marathon that will have a big impact on your future. Like training for a marathon, you'll need to start slowly and work your way up. When test day arrives, you'll be ready.

Start with the strategies you've read in the first two Secret Keys—plan your course and study in the way that works best for you. If you have time, consider using multiple study resources to get different approaches to the same concepts. It can be helpful to see difficult concepts from more than one angle. Then find a good source for practice tests. Many times, the test website will suggest potential study resources or provide sample tests.

Practice Test Strategy

If you're able to find at least three practice tests, we recommend this strategy:

UNTIMED AND OPEN-BOOK PRACTICE

Take the first test with no time constraints and with your notes and study guide handy. Take your time and focus on applying the strategies you've learned.

TIMED AND OPEN-BOOK PRACTICE

Take the second practice test open-book as well, but set a timer and practice pacing yourself to finish in time.

TIMED AND CLOSED-BOOK PRACTICE

Take any other practice tests as if it were test day. Set a timer and put away your study materials. Sit at a table or desk in a quiet room, imagine yourself at the testing center, and answer questions as quickly and accurately as possible.

Keep repeating timed and closed-book tests on a regular basis until you run out of practice tests or it's time for the actual test. Your mind will be ready for the schedule and stress of test day, and you'll be able to focus on recalling the material you've learned.

Secret Key #4 – Pace Yourself

Once you're fully prepared for the material on the test, your biggest challenge on test day will be managing your time. Just knowing that the clock is ticking can make you panic even if you have plenty of time left. Work on pacing yourself so you can build confidence against the time constraints of the exam. Pacing is a difficult skill to master, especially in a high-pressure environment, so **practice is vital**.

Set time expectations for your pace based on how much time is available. For example, if a section has 60 questions and the time limit is 30 minutes, you know you have to average 30 seconds or less per question in order to answer them all. Although 30 seconds is the hard limit, set 25 seconds per question as your goal, so you reserve extra time to spend on harder questions. When you budget extra time for the harder questions, you no longer have any reason to stress when those questions take longer to answer.

Don't let this time expectation distract you from working through the test at a calm, steady pace, but keep it in mind so you don't spend too much time on any one question. Recognize that taking extra time on one question you don't understand may keep you from answering two that you do understand later in the test. If your time limit for a question is up and you're still not sure of the answer, mark it and move on, and come back to it later if the time and the test format allow. If the testing format doesn't allow you to return to earlier questions, just make an educated guess; then put it out of your mind and move on.

On the easier questions, be careful not to rush. It may seem wise to hurry through them so you have more time for the challenging ones, but it's not worth missing one if you know the concept and just didn't take the time to read the question fully. Work efficiently but make sure you understand the question and have looked at all of the answer choices, since more than one may seem right at first.

Even if you're paying attention to the time, you may find yourself a little behind at some point. You should speed up to get back on track, but do so wisely. Don't panic; just take a few seconds less on each question until you're caught up. Don't guess without thinking, but do look through the answer choices and eliminate any you know are wrong. If you can get down to two choices, it is often worthwhile to guess from those. Once you've chosen an answer, move on and don't dwell on any that you skipped or had to hurry through. If a question was taking too long, chances are it was one of the harder ones, so you weren't as likely to get it right anyway.

On the other hand, if you find yourself getting ahead of schedule, it may be beneficial to slow down a little. The more quickly you work, the more likely you are to make a careless mistake that will affect your score. You've budgeted time for each question, so don't be afraid to spend that time. Practice an efficient but careful pace to get the most out of the time you have.

6

Secret Key #5 – Have a Plan for Guessing

When you're taking the test, you may find yourself stuck on a question. Some of the answer choices seem better than others, but you don't see the one answer choice that is obviously correct. What do you do?

The scenario described above is very common, yet most test takers have not effectively prepared for it. Developing and practicing a plan for guessing may be one of the single most effective uses of your time as you get ready for the exam.

In developing your plan for guessing, there are three questions to address:

- When should you start the guessing process?
- How should you narrow down the choices?
- Which answer should you choose?

When to Start the Guessing Process

Unless your plan for guessing is to select C every time (which, despite its merits, is not what we recommend), you need to leave yourself enough time to apply your answer elimination strategies. Since you have a limited amount of time for each question, that means that if you're going to give yourself the best shot at guessing correctly, you have to decide quickly whether or not you will guess.

Of course, the best-case scenario is that you don't have to guess at all, so first, see if you can answer the question based on your knowledge of the subject and basic reasoning skills. Focus on the key words in the question and try to jog your memory of related topics. Give yourself a chance to bring the knowledge to mind, but once you realize that you don't have (or you can't access) the knowledge you need to answer the question, it's time to start the guessing process.

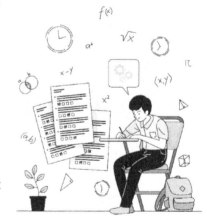

It's almost always better to start the guessing process too early than too late. It only takes a few seconds to remember something and answer the question from knowledge. Carefully eliminating wrong answer choices takes longer. Plus, going through the process of eliminating answer choices can actually help jog your memory.

Summary: Start the guessing process as soon as you decide that you can't answer the question based on your knowledge.

How to Narrow Down the Choices

The next chapter in this book (**Test-Taking Strategies**) includes a wide range of strategies for how to approach questions and how to look for answer choices to eliminate. You will definitely want to read those carefully, practice them, and figure out which ones work best for you. Here though, we're going to address a mindset rather than a particular strategy.

Your odds of guessing an answer correctly depend on how many options you are choosing from.

Number of options left	5	4	3	2	1
Odds of guessing correctly	20%	25%	33%	50%	100%

You can see from this chart just how valuable it is to be able to eliminate incorrect answers and make an educated guess, but there are two things that many test takers do that cause them to miss out on the benefits of guessing:

- Accidentally eliminating the correct answer
- Selecting an answer based on an impression

We'll look at the first one here, and the second one in the next section.

To avoid accidentally eliminating the correct answer, we recommend a thought exercise called **the $5 challenge**. In this challenge, you only eliminate an answer choice from contention if you are willing to bet $5 on it being wrong. Why $5? Five dollars is a small but not insignificant amount of money. It's an amount you could afford to lose but wouldn't want to throw away. And while losing

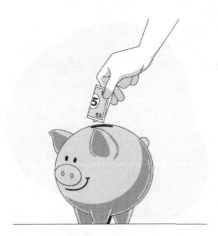

$5 once might not hurt too much, doing it twenty times will set you back $100. In the same way, each small decision you make—eliminating a choice here, guessing on a question there—won't by itself impact your score very much, but when you put them all together, they can make a big difference. By holding each answer choice elimination decision to a higher standard, you can reduce the risk of accidentally eliminating the correct answer.

The $5 challenge can also be applied in a positive sense: If you are willing to bet $5 that an answer choice *is* correct, go ahead and mark it as correct.

Summary: Only eliminate an answer choice if you are willing to bet $5 that it is wrong.

8

Which Answer to Choose

You're taking the test. You've run into a hard question and decided you'll have to guess. You've eliminated all the answer choices you're willing to bet $5 on. Now you have to pick an answer. Why do we even need to talk about this? Why can't you just pick whichever one you feel like when the time comes?

The answer to these questions is that if you don't come into the test with a plan, you'll rely on your impression to select an answer choice, and if you do that, you risk falling into a trap. The test writers know that everyone who takes their test will be guessing on some of the questions, so they intentionally write wrong answer choices to seem plausible. You still have to pick an answer though, and if the wrong answer choices are designed to look right, how can you ever be sure that you're not falling for their trap? The best solution we've found to this dilemma is to take the decision out of your hands entirely. Here is the process we recommend:

Once you've eliminated any choices that you are confident (willing to bet $5) are wrong, select the first remaining choice as your answer.

Whether you choose to select the first remaining choice, the second, or the last, the important thing is that you use some preselected standard. Using this approach guarantees that you will not be enticed into selecting an answer choice that looks right, because you are not basing your decision on how the answer choices look.

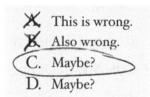

This is not meant to make you question your knowledge. Instead, it is to help you recognize the difference between your knowledge and your impressions. There's a huge difference between thinking an answer is right because of what you know, and thinking an answer is right because it looks or sounds like it should be right.

Summary: To ensure that your selection is appropriately random, make a predetermined selection from among all answer choices you have not eliminated.

Test-Taking Strategies

This section contains a list of test-taking strategies that you may find helpful as you work through the test. By taking what you know and applying logical thought, you can maximize your chances of answering any question correctly!

It is very important to realize that every question is different and every person is different: no single strategy will work on every question, and no single strategy will work for every person. That's why we've included all of them here, so you can try them out and determine which ones work best for different types of questions and which ones work best for you.

Question Strategies

☑ READ CAREFULLY

Read the question and the answer choices carefully. Don't miss the question because you misread the terms. You have plenty of time to read each question thoroughly and make sure you understand what is being asked. Yet a happy medium must be attained, so don't waste too much time. You must read carefully and efficiently.

☑ CONTEXTUAL CLUES

Look for contextual clues. If the question includes a word you are not familiar with, look at the immediate context for some indication of what the word might mean. Contextual clues can often give you all the information you need to decipher the meaning of an unfamiliar word. Even if you can't determine the meaning, you may be able to narrow down the possibilities enough to make a solid guess at the answer to the question.

☑ PREFIXES

If you're having trouble with a word in the question or answer choices, try dissecting it. Take advantage of every clue that the word might include. Prefixes can be a huge help. Usually, they allow you to determine a basic meaning. *Pre-* means before, *post-* means after, *pro-* is positive, *de-* is negative. From prefixes, you can get an idea of the general meaning of the word and try to put it into context.

☑ HEDGE WORDS

Watch out for critical hedge words, such as *likely*, *may*, *can*, *sometimes*, *often*, *almost*, *mostly*, *usually*, *generally*, *rarely*, and *sometimes*. Question writers insert these hedge phrases to cover every possibility. Often an answer choice will be wrong simply because it leaves no room for exception. Be on guard for answer choices that have definitive words such as *exactly* and *always*.

☑ SWITCHBACK WORDS

Stay alert for *switchbacks*. These are the words and phrases frequently used to alert you to shifts in thought. The most common switchback words are *but*, *although*, and *however*. Others include *nevertheless*, *on the other hand*, *even though*, *while*, *in spite of*, *despite*, and *regardless of*. Switchback words are important to catch because they can change the direction of the question or an answer choice.

⏀ FACE VALUE

When in doubt, use common sense. Accept the situation in the problem at face value. Don't read too much into it. These problems will not require you to make wild assumptions. If you have to go beyond creativity and warp time or space in order to have an answer choice fit the question, then you should move on and consider the other answer choices. These are normal problems rooted in reality. The applicable relationship or explanation may not be readily apparent, but it is there for you to figure out. Use your common sense to interpret anything that isn't clear.

Answer Choice Strategies

⏀ ANSWER SELECTION

The most thorough way to pick an answer choice is to identify and eliminate wrong answers until only one is left, then confirm it is the correct answer. Sometimes an answer choice may immediately seem right, but be careful. The test writers will usually put more than one reasonable answer choice on each question, so take a second to read all of them and make sure that the other choices are not equally obvious. As long as you have time left, it is better to read every answer choice than to pick the first one that looks right without checking the others.

⏀ ANSWER CHOICE FAMILIES

An answer choice family consists of two (in rare cases, three) answer choices that are very similar in construction and cannot all be true at the same time. If you see two answer choices that are direct opposites or parallels, one of them is usually the correct answer. For instance, if one answer choice says that quantity x increases and another either says that quantity x decreases (opposite) or says that quantity y increases (parallel), then those answer choices would fall into the same family. An answer choice that doesn't match the construction of the answer choice family is more likely to be incorrect. Most questions will not have answer choice families, but when they do appear, you should be prepared to recognize them.

⏀ ELIMINATE ANSWERS

Eliminate answer choices as soon as you realize they are wrong, but make sure you consider all possibilities. If you are eliminating answer choices and realize that the last one you are left with is also wrong, don't panic. Start over and consider each choice again. There may be something you missed the first time that you will realize on the second pass.

⏀ AVOID FACT TRAPS

Don't be distracted by an answer choice that is factually true but doesn't answer the question. You are looking for the choice that answers the question. Stay focused on what the question is asking for so you don't accidentally pick an answer that is true but incorrect. Always go back to the question and make sure the answer choice you've selected actually answers the question and is not merely a true statement.

⏀ EXTREME STATEMENTS

In general, you should avoid answers that put forth extreme actions as standard practice or proclaim controversial ideas as established fact. An answer choice that states the "process should be used in certain situations, if…" is much more likely to be correct than one that states the "process should be discontinued completely." The first is a calm rational statement and doesn't even make a definitive, uncompromising stance, using a hedge word *if* to provide wiggle room, whereas the second choice is far more extreme.

⊘ Benchmark

As you read through the answer choices and you come across one that seems to answer the question well, mentally select that answer choice. This is not your final answer, but it's the one that will help you evaluate the other answer choices. The one that you selected is your benchmark or standard for judging each of the other answer choices. Every other answer choice must be compared to your benchmark. That choice is correct until proven otherwise by another answer choice beating it. If you find a better answer, then that one becomes your new benchmark. Once you've decided that no other choice answers the question as well as your benchmark, you have your final answer.

⊘ Predict the Answer

Before you even start looking at the answer choices, it is often best to try to predict the answer. When you come up with the answer on your own, it is easier to avoid distractions and traps because you will know exactly what to look for. The right answer choice is unlikely to be word-for-word what you came up with, but it should be a close match. Even if you are confident that you have the right answer, you should still take the time to read each option before moving on.

General Strategies

⊘ Tough Questions

If you are stumped on a problem or it appears too hard or too difficult, don't waste time. Move on! Remember though, if you can quickly check for obviously incorrect answer choices, your chances of guessing correctly are greatly improved. Before you completely give up, at least try to knock out a couple of possible answers. Eliminate what you can and then guess at the remaining answer choices before moving on.

⊘ Check Your Work

Since you will probably not know every term listed and the answer to every question, it is important that you get credit for the ones that you do know. Don't miss any questions through careless mistakes. If at all possible, try to take a second to look back over your answer selection and make sure you've selected the correct answer choice and haven't made a costly careless mistake (such as marking an answer choice that you didn't mean to mark). This quick double check should more than pay for itself in caught mistakes for the time it costs.

⊘ Pace Yourself

It's easy to be overwhelmed when you're looking at a page full of questions; your mind is confused and full of random thoughts, and the clock is ticking down faster than you would like. Calm down and maintain the pace that you have set for yourself. Especially as you get down to the last few minutes of the test, don't let the small numbers on the clock make you panic. As long as you are on track by monitoring your pace, you are guaranteed to have time for each question.

⊘ Don't Rush

It is very easy to make errors when you are in a hurry. Maintaining a fast pace in answering questions is pointless if it makes you miss questions that you would have gotten right otherwise. Test writers like to include distracting information and wrong answers that seem right. Taking a little extra time to avoid careless mistakes can make all the difference in your test score. Find a pace that allows you to be confident in the answers that you select.

⊘ Keep Moving

Panicking will not help you pass the test, so do your best to stay calm and keep moving. Taking deep breaths and going through the answer elimination steps you practiced can help to break through a stress barrier and keep your pace.

Final Notes

The combination of a solid foundation of content knowledge and the confidence that comes from practicing your plan for applying that knowledge is the key to maximizing your performance on test day. As your foundation of content knowledge is built up and strengthened, you'll find that the strategies included in this chapter become more and more effective in helping you quickly sift through the distractions and traps of the test to isolate the correct answer.

Now that you're preparing to move forward into the test content chapters of this book, be sure to keep your goal in mind. As you read, think about how you will be able to apply this information on the test. If you've already seen sample questions for the test and you have an idea of the question format and style, try to come up with questions of your own that you can answer based on what you're reading. This will give you valuable practice applying your knowledge in the same ways you can expect to on test day.

Good luck and good studying!

Anatomy and Physiology

Structure and Function

TISSUES

Tissues are groups of cells that work together to perform a specific function. Tissues can be grouped into four broad categories: muscle tissue, nerve tissue, epithelial tissue, and connective tissue.

CATEGORIES

The categories of tissues are as follows:

- **Epithelial** – Tissue in which cells are joined together tightly. Skin tissue is an example.
- **Connective** – Connective tissue may be dense, loose or fatty. It protects and binds body parts. Connective tissues include bone tissue, cartilage, tendons, ligaments, fat, blood, and lymph.
- **Cartilage** – Cushions and provides structural support for body parts. It has a jelly-like base and is fibrous.
- **Blood** – Blood transports oxygen to cells and removes wastes. It also carries hormones and defends against disease.
- **Bone** – Bone is a hard tissue that supports and protects softer tissues and organs. Its marrow produces red blood cells.
- **Muscle** – Muscle tissue helps support and move the body. The three types of muscle tissue are smooth, cardiac, and skeletal.
- **Nervous** – Nerve tissue is located in the brain, spinal cord, and nerves. Cells called neurons form a network through the body that control responses to changes in the external and internal environment. Some send signals to muscles and glands to trigger responses.

ORGANS

Organs are groups of tissues that work together to perform specific functions.

ORGANS GROUPED IN MULTIPLE SYSTEMS

Complex animals have several organs that are grouped together in multiple systems. For example, the heart is specifically designed to pump blood throughout an organism's body. The heart is composed mostly of muscle tissue in the myocardium, but it also contains connective tissue in the blood and membranes, nervous tissue that controls the heart rate, and epithelial tissue in the membranes. Gills in fish and lungs in reptiles, birds, and mammals are specifically designed to exchange gases. In birds, crops are designed to store food and gizzards are designed to grind food.

MAJOR ORGAN SYSTEMS

In mammals, there are 11 major organ systems: integumentary system, respiratory system, cardiovascular system, endocrine system, nervous system, immune system, digestive system, excretory system, muscular system, skeletal system, and reproductive system.

BODY PLANES

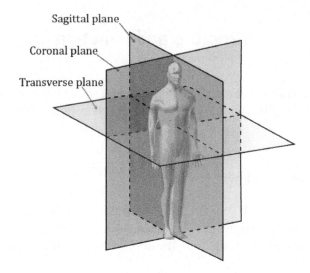

Sagittal plane

Coronal plane

Transverse plane

The three primary body planes are discussed below:

- The *Transverse (or horizontal) plane* divides the patient's body into imaginary upper (superior) and lower (inferior or caudal) halves.
- The *Sagittal plane* divides the body, or any body part, vertically into right and left sections. The sagittal plane runs parallel to the midline of the body.
- The *Coronal (or frontal) plane* divides the body, or any body structure, vertically into front and back (anterior and posterior) sections. The coronal plane runs vertically through the body at right angles to the midline.

TERMS OF DIRECTION

Terms of direction are defined below:

- *Medial* means nearer to the midline of the body. In anatomical position, the little finger is medial to the thumb.
- *Lateral* is the opposite of medial. It refers to structures further away from the body's midline, at the sides. In anatomical position, the thumb is lateral to the little finger.
- *Proximal* refers to structures closer to the center of the body. The hip is proximal to the knee.
- *Distal* refers to structures further away from the center of the body. The knee is distal to the hip.
- *Anterior* refers to structures in front.
- *Posterior* refers to structures behind.
- *Superior* means above, or closer to the head.
- *Inferior* means below, or closer to the feet.
- *Cephalad* and cephalic are adverbs meaning towards the head. Cranial is the adjective, meaning of the skull.
- *Caudad* is an adverb meaning towards the tail or posterior. Caudal is the adjective, meaning of the hindquarters.

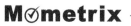

CIRCULATORY SYSTEM
RESPONSIBILITY AND MAIN PARTS

The circulatory system is responsible for the internal transport of substances to and from the cells. The circulatory system usually consists of the following three parts:

- **Blood** – Blood is composed of water, solutes, and other elements in a fluid connective tissue.
- **Blood Vessels** – Tubules of different sizes that transport blood.
- **Heart** – The heart is a muscular pump providing the pressure necessary to keep blood flowing.

OPEN OR CLOSED CIRCULATORY SYSTEM

Circulatory systems can be either open or closed. Most animals have closed systems, where the heart and blood vessels are continually connected.

RATE OF BLOOD FLOW

As the blood moves through the system from larger tubules through smaller ones, the rate slows down. The flow of blood in the capillary beds, the smallest tubules, is quite slow.

PURPOSE AND AMOUNT OF BLOOD IN AVERAGE ADULT HUMAN

Blood helps maintain a healthy internal environment in animals by carrying raw materials to cells and removing waste products. It helps stabilize internal pH and hosts cells of the immune system.

An adult human has about five quarts of blood. Blood is composed of **red blood cells, white blood cells**, **platelets**, and **plasma**. Plasma constitutes more than half of the blood volume. It is mostly water and serves as a solvent. Plasma contains plasma proteins, ions, glucose, amino acids, hormones, and dissolved gases. **Platelets** are fragments of stem cells and serve an important function in blood clotting.

Red blood cells transport **oxygen** to cells. Red blood cells form in the bone marrow and can live for about four months. These cells are constantly being replaced by fresh ones, keeping the total number relatively stable. They lack a nucleus.

Part of the immune system, white blood cells defend the body against **infection** and remove wastes. The types of white blood cells include lymphocytes, neutrophils, monocytes, eosinophils, and basophils.

HEART

The **heart** is a muscular pump made of cardiac muscle tissue. Heart chamber contraction and relaxation is coordinated by electrical signals from the self-exciting **sinoatrial node** and the **atrioventricular node**. **Atrial contraction** fills the ventricles and **ventricular contraction** forces blood into arteries leaving the heart. This sequence is called the **cardiac cycle**. Valves keep blood moving through the heart in a single direction and prevent any backwash as it flows through its four chambers.

Deoxygenated blood from the body flows through the heart in this order:

1. The **superior vena cava** brings blood from the upper body; the **inferior vena cava** brings blood from the lower body.
2. Right atrium
3. Tricuspid valve (right atrioventricular [AV] valve)

17

4. Right ventricle
5. Pulmonary valve
6. Left and right pulmonary artery (note: these arteries carry deoxygenated blood)
7. Lungs (where gas exchange occurs)

Oxygenated blood returns to the body through:

1. Left and right pulmonary veins (note: these veins carry oxygenated blood)
2. Left atrium
3. Mitral valve (left atrioventricular [AV] valve)
4. Left ventricle
5. Aortic valve
6. Aortic arch
7. Aorta

The left and right sides of the heart are separated by the septum. The heart has its own circulatory system with its own **coronary arteries**.

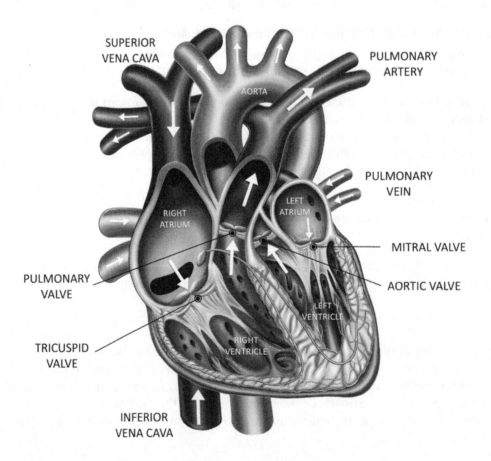

Review Video: Heart Blood Flow and Heart Anatomy
Visit mometrix.com/academy and enter code: 783139

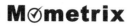

Anatomy and Physiology

CARDIAC CYCLE

The heart functions by contracting and relaxing. Atrial contraction fills the ventricles and ventricular contraction empties them, forcing circulation. This sequence is called the cardiac cycle. The cardiac cycle consists of diastole and systole phases, which can be further divided into the first and second phases to describe the events of the right and left sides of the heart. However, these events are simultaneously occurring.

COMPLEX ELECTRICAL SYSTEM

Cardiac muscles are attached to each other and signals for contractions spread rapidly. A complex electrical system controls the heartbeat as cardiac muscle cells produce and conduct electric signals. These muscles are said to be self-exciting, needing no external stimuli.

MOVEMENT OF BLOOD FROM THE SUPERIOR AND INFERIOR VENAE CAVAE TO THE RIGHT VENTRICLE

During the first diastole phase, blood flows through the superior and inferior venae cavae. Because the heart is relaxed, blood flows passively from the atrium through the open atrioventricular valve (tricuspid valve) to the right ventricle. The sinoatrial (SA) node, the cardiac pacemaker located in the wall of the right atrium, generates electrical signals, which are carried by the Purkinje fibers to the rest of the atrium, stimulating it to contract and fill the right ventricle with blood.

INITIATION OF FIRST SYSTOLE PHASE

The impulse from the SA node is transmitted to the ventricle through the atrioventricular (AV) node, signaling the right ventricle to contract and initiating the first systole phase.

TIME BETWEEN THE TRICUSPID VALVE CLOSING AND BLOOD FILLING THE LEFT VENTRICLE

The tricuspid valve closes, and the pulmonary semilunar valve opens. Blood is pumped out the pulmonary arteries to the lungs. Blood returning from the lungs fills the left atrium as part of the second diastole phase. The SA node triggers the mitral valve to open, and blood fills the left ventricle.

SECOND SYSTOLE PHASE

During the second systole phase, the mitral valve closes and the aortic semilunar valve opens. The left ventricle contracts, and blood is pumped out of the aorta to the rest of the body.

TYPES OF CIRCULATION IN CIRCULATORY SYSTEM

The circulatory system includes coronary circulation, pulmonary circulation, and systemic circulation.

- **Coronary Circulation** - Coronary circulation is the flow of blood to the heart tissue. Blood enters the coronary arteries, which branch off the aorta, supplying major arteries, which enter the heart with oxygenated blood. The deoxygenated blood returns to the right atrium through the cardiac veins, which empty into the coronary sinus.
- **Pulmonary Circulation** - Pulmonary circulation is the flow of blood between the heart and the lungs. Deoxygenated blood flows from the right ventricle to the lungs through pulmonary arteries. Oxygenated blood flows back to the left atrium through the pulmonary veins.

19

- **Systemic Circulation** - Systemic circulation is the flow of blood to the entire body with the exception of coronary circulation and pulmonary circulation. Blood exits the left ventricle through the aorta, which branches into the carotid arteries, subclavian arteries, common iliac arteries, and the renal artery. Blood returns to the heart through the jugular veins, subclavian veins, common iliac veins, and renal veins, which empty into the superior and inferior venae cavae.
- **Portal Circulation** - Included in systemic circulation is portal circulation, which is the flow of blood from the digestive system to the liver and then to the heart, and renal circulation, which is the flow of blood between the heart and the kidneys.

BLOOD PRESSURE, ARTERIAL BLOOD PRESSURE, ARTERIES, AND ARTERIOLES

Blood pressure is the fluid pressure generated by the cardiac cycle. Arterial blood pressure functions by transporting oxygen-poor blood into the lungs and oxygen-rich blood to the body tissues. Arteries branch into smaller arterioles which contract and expand based on signals from the body. Arterioles are where adjustments are made in blood delivery to specific areas based on complex communication from body systems.

CAPILLARY BEDS AND CAPILLARIES

Capillary beds are diffusion sites for exchanges between blood and interstitial fluid. A capillary has the thinnest wall of any blood vessel, consisting of a single layer of endothelial cells.

VEINS

Capillaries merge into venules which in turn merge with larger diameter tubules called veins. Veins transport blood from body tissues back to the heart. Valves inside the veins facilitate this transport. The walls of veins are thin and contain smooth muscle and also function as blood volume reserves.

DIGESTIVE SYSTEM

FUNCTIONS

The digestive system uses the following processes to convert protein, fats, and carbohydrates into usable energy for the body:

- **Movement**: Movement mixes and passes nutrients through the system and eliminates waste.
- **Secretion**: Enzymes, hormones, and other substances necessary for digestion are secreted into the digestive tract.
- **Digestion**: Digestion includes the chemical breakdown of nutrients into smaller units that enter the internal environment.
- **Absorption**: Nutrients pass through plasma membranes into the blood or lymph and then to the body.

> **Review Video: Gastrointestinal System**
> Visit mometrix.com/academy and enter code: 378740

CONTENTS

The human digestive system consists of the mouth, pharynx, esophagus, stomach, small and large intestine, rectum, and anus.

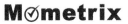

ROLE OF THE MOUTH

Digestion begins in the mouth with the chewing and mixing of nutrients with saliva. Salivary glands are stimulated and secrete saliva. Saliva contains enzymes that initiate the breakdown of starch in digestion. Once swallowed, the food moves down the pharynx into the esophagus en route to the stomach. Only humans and other mammals actually chew their food.

FUNCTIONS OF THE STOMACH

As a flexible, muscular sac, the stomach has three main functions:

- Mixing and storing food
- Dissolving and degrading food via secretions
- Controlling passage of food into the small intestine

RESPONSIBILITY OF STOMACH ACIDITY AND ROLE OF SMOOTH MUSCLE CONTRACTIONS

Protein digestion begins in the stomach. Stomach acidity helps break down the food and make nutrients available for absorption. Smooth muscle moves the food by peristalsis, contracting and relaxing to move nutrients along. Smooth muscle contractions move nutrients into the small intestine where the absorption process begins.

SMALL INTESTINE

ROLE OF ENZYMES AND BILE IN DIGESTION IN THE SMALL INTESTINE

Enzymes from the pancreas, liver, and stomach are transported to the small intestine to aid digestion. These enzymes act on fats, carbohydrates, nucleic acids, and proteins. Bile is a secretion of the liver and is particularly useful in breaking down fats. It is stored in the gall bladder between meals.

VILLI

By the time food reaches the lining of the small intestine, it has been reduced to small molecules. The lining of the small intestine is covered with villi, tiny absorptive structures that greatly increase the surface area for interaction with chyme (the semi-liquid mass of partially digested food). Epithelial cells at the surface of the villi, called microvilli, further increase the ability of the small intestine to serve as the main absorption organ of the digestive tract.

LARGE INTESTINE

Also called the colon, the large intestine concentrates, mixes, and stores waste material. A little over a meter in length, the colon ascends on the right side of the abdominal cavity, cuts across transversely to the left side, then descends and attaches to the rectum, a short tube for waste disposal.

EXPELLING OF WASTE

When the rectal wall is distended by waste material, the nervous system triggers an impulse in the body to expel the waste from the rectum. A muscle sphincter at the end of the anus is stimulated to facilitate the expelling of waste matter.

SPEED AT WHICH WASTE MOVES THROUGH THE LARGE INTESTINE

The speed at which waste moves through the colon is influenced by the volume of fiber and other undigested material present. Without adequate bulk in the diet, it takes longer to move waste along, sometimes with negative effects. Lack of bulk in the diet has been linked to a number of disorders.

PANCREAS

The pancreas is six to ten inches long in an adult and located at the back of the abdomen behind the stomach. It is a long, tapered organ. The wider (right) side is called the **head,** and the narrower (left) side is called the **tail**. The head lies near the **duodenum** (the first section of the small intestine), and the tail ends near the **spleen**. The body of the pancreas lies between the head and the tail. The pancreas is made up of exocrine and endocrine tissues. The **exocrine tissue** secretes digestive enzymes from a series of ducts that collectively form the main pancreatic duct (that runs the length of the pancreas). The **main pancreatic duct** connects to the common bile duct near the duodenum. The **endocrine tissue** secretes hormones (such as insulin) into the bloodstream. Blood is supplied to the pancreas from the splenic artery, gastroduodenal artery, and superior mesenteric artery.

EXOCRINE TISSUES AND ENDOCRINE TISSUE

The pancreas is made up of exocrine and endocrine tissues. The exocrine tissue secretes digestive enzymes from a series of ducts that collectively form the main pancreatic duct (that runs the length of the pancreas). The main pancreatic duct connects to the common bile duct near the duodenum. The endocrine tissue secretes hormones (such as insulin) into the bloodstream.

BLOOD SUPPLY TO THE PANCREAS

Blood is supplied to the pancreas from the splenic artery, gastroduodenal artery, and the superior mesenteric artery.

ASSISTANCE IN DIGESTION

The pancreas assists in the digestion of foods by secreting enzymes (to the small intestine) that help to break down many foods, especially fats and proteins.

ENZYMES SECRETED BY THE PANCREAS

The precursors to these enzymes (called zymogens) are produced by groups of exocrine cells (called acini). They are converted, through a chemical reaction in the gut, to the active enzymes (such as pancreatic lipase and amylase) once they enter the small intestine.

SECRETION OF SODIUM BICARBONATE

The pancreas also secretes large amounts of sodium bicarbonate to neutralize the stomach acid that reaches the small intestine.

EXOCRINE FUNCTIONS

The exocrine functions of the pancreas are controlled by hormones released by the stomach and small intestine (duodenum) when food is present. The exocrine secretions of the pancreas flow into the main pancreatic duct (Wirsung's duct) and are delivered to the duodenum through the pancreatic duct.

ENDOCRINE SYSTEM

The endocrine system is responsible for secreting **hormones** and other molecules that help regulate the entire body in both the short and long term. There is a close working relationship between the endocrine and nervous systems. The **hypothalamus** and the **pituitary gland** coordinate to serve as a **neuroendocrine control center**.

Hormone secretion is triggered by a variety of signals, including hormonal signs, chemical reactions, and environmental cues. Only cells with particular **receptors** can benefit from hormonal influence. This is the "key in the lock" model for hormonal action. **Steroid hormones** trigger gene activation and protein synthesis in some target cells. **Protein hormones** change the activity of existing enzymes in target cells. Hormones such as **insulin** work quickly when the body signals an urgent need. Slower-acting hormones afford longer, gradual, and sometimes permanent changes in the body.

TRIGGER OF HORMONE SECRETION

Hormone secretion is triggered by a variety of signals, including hormonal signs, chemical reactions, and environmental cues.

KEY IN THE LOCK MODEL FOR HORMONAL ACTION

Only cells with particular receptors can benefit from hormonal influence. This is the "key in the lock" model for hormonal action.

ROLE OF STEROID AND PROTEIN HORMONES

Steroid hormones trigger gene activation and protein synthesis in some target cells. Protein hormones change the activity of existing enzymes in target cells.

QUICK-ACTING AND SLOW-ACTING HORMONES

Hormones such as insulin work quickly when the body signals an urgent need. Slower acting hormones afford longer, gradual, and sometimes permanent changes in the body.

MAJOR ENDOCRINE GLANDS

The eight major endocrine glands and their functions are:

- **Adrenal cortex** – Monitors blood sugar level; helps in lipid and protein metabolism.
- **Adrenal medulla** – Controls cardiac function; raises blood sugar and controls the size of blood vessels.
- **Thyroid gland** – Helps regulate metabolism and functions in growth and development.
- **Parathyroid** – Regulates calcium levels in the blood.
- **Pancreas islets** – Raises and lowers blood sugar; active in carbohydrate metabolism.
- **Thymus gland** – Plays a role in immune responses.
- **Pineal gland** – Has an influence on daily biorhythms and sexual activity.
- **Pituitary gland** – Plays an important role in growth and development.

ISLETS OF LANGERHANS

Located amongst the groupings of exocrine cells (acini) are groups of endocrine cells (called islets of Langerhans). The islets of Langerhans are primarily made up of insulin-producing beta cells (fifty to eighty percent of the total) and glucagon-releasing alpha cells.

INSULIN AND GLUCAGON

The major hormones produced by the pancreas are insulin and glucagon. The body uses insulin to control carbohydrate metabolism by lowering the amount of sugar (glucose) in the blood. Insulin also affects fat metabolism and can change the liver's ability to release stored fat. The body also uses glucagon to control carbohydrate metabolism. Glucagon has the opposite effect of insulin in that the body uses it to increase blood sugar (glucose) levels. The levels of insulin and glucagon are balanced to maintain the optimum level of blood sugar (glucose) throughout the day.

THYROID GLAND AND PARATHYROID GLAND

The thyroid and parathyroid glands are located in the neck just below the larynx. The parathyroid glands are four small glands that are embedded on the posterior side of the thyroid gland. The basic function of the thyroid gland is to regulate metabolism. The thyroid gland secretes the hormones thyroxine, triiodothyronine, and calcitonin. Thyroxine and triiodothyronine increase metabolism, and calcitonin decreases blood calcium by storing calcium in bone tissue.

HYPOTHALAMUS AND PARATHYROID GLANDS

The hypothalamus directs the pituitary gland to secrete thyroid-stimulating hormone (TSH), which stimulates the thyroid gland to release these hormones as needed via a negative-feedback mechanism. The parathyroid glands secrete parathyroid hormone, which can increase blood calcium by moving calcium from the bone to the blood.

INTEGUMENTARY SYSTEM

The integumentary system, which consists of the skin including the sebaceous glands, sweat glands, hair, and nails, serves a variety of functions associated with protection, secretion, and communication. In the functions associated with protection, the integumentary system protects the body from **pathogens** including bacteria, viruses, and chemicals. In the functions associated with secretion, **sebaceous glands** secrete **sebum** (oil) that waterproofs the skin, and **sweat glands** assist with **thermoregulation**. Sweat glands also serve as excretory organs and help rid the body of metabolic waste. In the functions associated with communication, **sensory receptors** distributed throughout the skin send information to the brain regarding pain, touch, pressure, and temperature. In addition to protection, secretion, and communication, the skin manufactures **vitamin D** with the help of ultraviolet light and can absorb certain chemicals, such as specific medications.

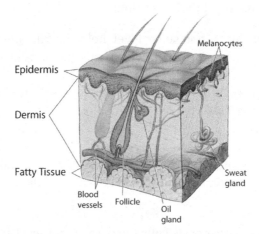

FUNCTIONS ASSOCIATED WITH PROTECTION, SECRETION, AND COMMUNICATION

In the functions associated with protection, the integumentary system protects the body from pathogens including bacteria, viruses, and various chemicals from entering the body. In the functions associated with secretion, sebaceous glands secrete sebum (oil) that waterproofs the skin, and sweat glands are associated with the body's homeostatic relationship of thermoregulation. Sweat glands also serve as excretory organs and help rid the body of metabolic wastes. In the functions associated with communication, sensory receptors distributed throughout the skin send information to the brain regarding pain, touch, pressure, and temperature.

> **Review Video: Integumentary System**
> Visit mometrix.com/academy and enter code: 655980

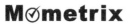

Anatomy and Physiology

VITAMIN D AND CHEMICALS

In addition to protection, secretion, and communication, the skin manufactures vitamin D and can absorb certain chemicals such as specific medications.

LAYERS

The layers of the skin from the surface of the skin inward are the epidermis and dermis. The subcutaneous layer lying below the dermis is also part of the integumentary system. The epidermis is the most superficial layer of the skin. The epidermis, which consists entirely of epithelial cells, does not contain any blood vessels. The deepest portion of the epidermis is the stratum basale, which is a single layer of cells that continually undergo division.

RENEWAL OF SKIN CELLS

As more and more cells are produced, older cells are pushed toward the surface. Most epidermal cells are keratinized. Keratin is a waxy protein that helps to waterproof the skin. As the cells die, they are sloughed off.

DERMIS

The dermis lies directly beneath the epidermis. The dermis consists mostly of connective tissue. The dermis contains blood vessels, sensory receptors, hair follicles, sebaceous glands, and sweat glands. The dermis also contains elastin and collagen fibers.

SUBCUTANEOUS LAYER

The subcutaneous layer or hypodermis is actually not a layer of the skin. The subcutaneous layer consists of connective tissue, which binds the skin to the underlying muscles. Fat deposits in the subcutaneous layer help to cushion and insulate the body.

TEMPERATURE HOMEOSTASIS

The skin is involved in temperature homeostasis or thermoregulation through the activation of the sweat glands. By thermoregulation, the body maintains a stable body temperature as one component of a stable internal environment. The temperature of the body is controlled by a negative feedback system consisting of a receptor, control center, and effector. The receptors are sensory cells located in the dermis of the skin. The control center is the hypothalamus, which is located in the brain. The effectors include the sweat glands, blood vessels, and muscles. The evaporation of sweat across the surface of the skin cools the body to maintain its tolerance range. Vasodilation of the blood vessels near the surface of the skin also releases heat into the environment to lower body temperature. The muscles that are included with the effectors are partly responsible for shivering which is also associated with the muscular system.

EXOCRINE GLANDS

Sebaceous glands and sweat glands are exocrine glands found in the skin. Exocrine glands secrete substances into ducts. In this case, the secretions are through the ducts to the surface of the skin.

SEBACEOUS GLANDS AND SEBUM

Sebaceous glands are holocrine glands, which secrete sebum. Sebum is an oily mixture of lipids and proteins. Sebaceous glands are connected to hair follicles and secrete sebum through the hair pore. Sebum inhibits water loss from the skin and protects against bacterial and fungal infections.

SWEAT GLANDS

ECCRINE GLANDS

Sweat glands are either eccrine glands or apocrine glands. Eccrine glands are not connected to hair follicles. They are activated by elevated body temperature. Eccrine glands are located throughout the body and can be found on the forehead, neck, and back. Eccrine glands secrete a salty solution of electrolytes and water containing sodium chloride, potassium, bicarbonate, glucose, and antimicrobial peptides. Eccrine glands are activated as part of the body's thermoregulation.

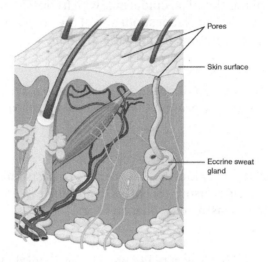

APOCRINE GLANDS

Apocrine glands secrete an oily solution containing fatty acids, triglycerides, and proteins. Apocrine glands are located in the armpits, groin, palms, and soles of the feet. Apocrine glands secrete this oily sweat when a person experiences stress or anxiety. Bacteria feed on apocrine sweat and expel aromatic fatty acids, producing body odor.

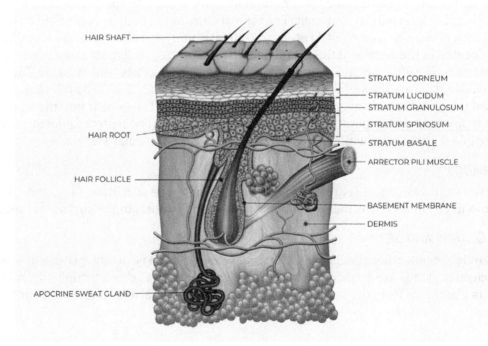

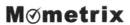

Anatomy and Physiology

LYMPHATIC SYSTEM

The main function of the lymphatic system is to return excess tissue fluid to the bloodstream. This system consists of transport vessels and lymphoid organs. The lymph vascular system consists of lymph capillaries, lymph vessels, and lymph ducts.

FUNCTIONS OF THE LYMPH VASCULAR SYSTEM

The major functions of the lymph vascular system are:

- The return of excess fluid to the blood.
- The return of protein from the capillaries.
- The transport of fats from the digestive tract.
- The disposal of debris and cellular waste.

LYMPHOID ORGANS

Lymphoid organs include the lymph nodes, spleen, appendix, adenoids, thymus, tonsils, and small patches of tissue in the small intestine.

LYMPH NODES

Lymph nodes are located at intervals throughout the lymph vessel system. Each node contains lymphocytes and plasma cells.

THYMUS

The thymus secretes hormones and is the major site of lymphocyte production.

SPLEEN

The spleen stores macrophages which help to filter red blood cells. The spleen is in the upper left of the abdomen. It is located behind the stomach and immediately below the diaphragm. It is about the size of a thick paperback book and weighs just over half a pound. It is made up of lymphoid tissue. The blood vessels are connected to the spleen by splenic sinuses (modified capillaries). The main functions of the spleen are to filter unwanted materials from the blood (including old red blood cells) and to help fight infections. The following peritoneal ligaments support the spleen:

- The gastrolienal ligament that connects the stomach to the spleen.
- The lienorenal ligament that connects the kidney to the spleen.
- The middle section of the phrenicocolic ligament (connects the left colic flexure to the thoracic diaphragm).

MUSCLES

COMMON PROPERTIES

All muscles have these three properties in common:

- **Excitability** – All muscle tissues have an electric gradient which can reverse when stimulated.
- **Contraction** – All muscle tissues have the ability to contract, or shorten.
- **Elongate** – All muscle tissues share the capacity to elongate, or relax.

VOLUNTARY MUSCLE

Skeletal muscles are voluntary muscles that work in pairs to move various parts of the skeleton. Skeletal muscles are composed of muscle fibers (cells) that are bound together in parallel bundles.

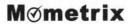

Skeletal muscles are also known as striated muscle due to their striped appearance under a microscope.

INVOLUNTARY MUSCLES

Smooth muscle tissues are involuntary muscles that are found in the walls of internal organs such as the stomach, intestines, and blood vessels. Smooth muscle tissues or visceral tissue is nonstriated. Smooth muscle cells are shorter and wider than skeletal muscle fibers. Smooth muscle tissue is also found in sphincters or valves that control various openings throughout the body. Cardiac muscle tissue is involuntary muscle that is found only in the heart. Like skeletal muscle cells, cardiac muscle cells are also striated.

INTERACTION OF THE SKELETON AND SKELETAL MUSCLE

Only skeletal muscle interacts with the skeleton to move the body. When they contract, the muscles transmit force to the attached bones. Working together, the muscles and bones act as a system of levers which move around the joints. A small contraction of a muscle can produce a large movement. A limb can be extended and rotated around a joint due to the way the muscles are arranged.

COMPOSITION OF SKELETAL MUSCLES AND MUSCLE FIBERS

Skeletal muscles consist of numerous muscle fibers. Each muscle fiber contains a bundle of myofibrils, which are composed of multiple repeating contractile units called sarcomeres.

PROTEIN MICROFILAMENTS OF MYOFIBRILS AND TYPES OF STRIATIONS IN SKELETAL MUSCLES

Myofibrils contain two protein microfilaments: a thick filament and a thin filament. The thick filament is composed of the protein myosin. The thin filament is composed of the protein actin. The dark bands (striations) in skeletal muscles are formed when thick and thin filaments overlap. Light bands occur where the thin filament is overlapped. Skeletal muscle attraction occurs when the thin filaments slide over the thick filaments shortening the sarcomere.

SLIDING FILAMENT MODEL OF MUSCLE CONTRACTION

When an action potential (electrical signal) reaches a muscle fiber, calcium ions are released. According to the sliding filament model of muscle contraction, these calcium ions bind to the myosin and actin, which assists in the binding of the myosin heads of the thick filaments to the actin molecules of the thin filaments. Adenosine triphosphate released from glucose provides the energy necessary for the contraction.

HUMAN NERVOUS SYSTEM

The human nervous system senses, interprets, and issues commands as a response to conditions in the body's environment. This process is made possible by a complex communication system of cells called **neurons**.

Messages are sent across the plasma membrane of neurons through a process called **action potential**. These messages occur when a neuron is stimulated past a necessary threshold. These stimulations occur in a sequence from the stimulation point of one neuron to its contact with another neuron. At the point of contact, called a **chemical synapse**, a substance is released that stimulates or inhibits the action of the adjoining cell. A network of nerves composed of neurons

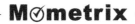

fans out across the body and forms the framework for the nervous system. The direction the information flows depends on the specific organizations of nerve circuits and pathways.

> **Review Video: <u>What is the Function of the Nervous System</u>**
> Visit mometrix.com/academy and enter code: 708428

Anatomy and Physiology

SENSORY NEURONS, MOTOR NEURONS, AND INTERNEURONS

Sensory neurons transmit signals to the central nervous system (CNS) from the sensory receptors associated with touch, pain, temperature, hearing, sight, smell, and taste. Motor neurons transmit signals from the CNS to the rest of the body such as by signaling muscles or glands to respond. Interneurons transmit signals between neurons; for example, interneurons receive transmitted signals between sensory neurons and motor neurons.

DENDRITES, CELL BODY, AND AXON

The dendrites receive impulses from sensory receptors or interneurons and transmit them toward the cell body. The cell body (soma) contains the nucleus of the neuron. The axon transmits the impulses away from the cell body. The axon is insulated by oligodendrocytes and the myelin sheath with gaps known as the nodes of Ranvier. The axon terminates at the synapse.

SPINAL CORD

The spinal cord is encased in the bony structure of the vertebrae, which protects and supports it. Its nervous tissue functions mainly with respect to limb movement and internal organ activity. Major nerve tracts ascend and descend from the spinal cord to the brain.

FRONTAL AND PARIETAL LOBES IN THE BRAIN

The frontal lobe located in the front of the brain is responsible for a short term and working memory and information processing as well as decision-making, planning, and judgment. The parietal lobe is located slightly toward the back of the brain and the top of the head and is responsible for sensory input as well as spatial positioning of the body.

OCCIPITAL AND TEMPORAL LOBES IN THE BRAIN

The occipital lobe is located at the back of the head just above the brain stem. This lobe is responsible for visual input, processing, and output; specifically nerves from the eyes enter directly into this lobe. Finally, the temporal lobes are located at the left and right sides of the brain. These lobes are responsible for all auditory input, processing, and output.

CEREBELLUM

The cerebellum plays a role in the processing and storing of implicit memories. Specifically, for those memories developed during classical conditioning learning techniques. The role of the cerebellum was discovered by exploring the memory of individuals with damaged cerebellums. These individuals were unable to develop stimulus responses when presented via a classical conditioning technique. Researchers found that this was also the case for automatic responses. For example, when these individuals were presented with a puff or air into their eyes, they did not blink, which would have been the naturally occurring and automatic response in an individual with no brain damage.

BRAIN STEM

The posterior area of the brain that is connected to the spinal cord is known as the brain stem. The midbrain, the pons, and the medulla oblongata are the three parts of the brain stem. Information from the body is sent to the brain through the brain stem, and information from the brain is sent to

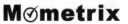

the body through the brain stem. The brain stem is an important part of respiratory, digestive, and circulatory functions.

MIDBRAIN

The midbrain lies above the pons and the medulla oblongata. The parts of the midbrain include the tectum, the tegmentum, and the ventral tegmentum.

PONS AND MEDULLA OBLONGATA

The pons comes between the midbrain and the medulla oblongata. Information is sent across the pons from the cerebrum to the medulla and the cerebellum. The medulla oblongata (or medulla) is beneath the midbrain and the pons. The medulla oblongata is the piece of the brain stem that connects the spinal cord to the brain. The medulla oblongata has an important role with the autonomous nervous system in the circulatory and respiratory system.

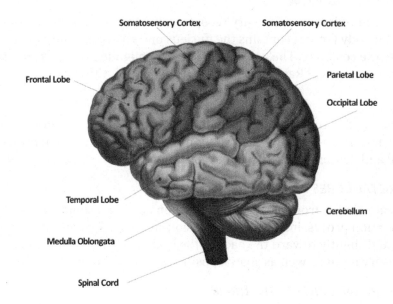

PERIPHERAL NERVOUS SYSTEM

The **peripheral nervous system** consists of the nerves and ganglia throughout the body that control both voluntary movement and involuntary functions. Involuntary functions are managed by **sympathetic nerves,** which trigger the "fight or flight" response, and **parasympathetic nerves,** which control basic "rest and digest" body functions.

ANS

The autonomic nervous system (ANS) maintains homeostasis within the body. In general, the ANS controls the functions of the internal organs, blood vessels, smooth muscle tissues, and glands. This is accomplished through the direction of the hypothalamus, which is located above the midbrain. The hypothalamus controls the ANS through the brain stem. With this direction from the hypothalamus, the ANS helps maintain a stable body environment (homeostasis) by regulating numerous factors including heart rate, breathing rate, body temperature, and blood pH.

DIVISIONS AND ROLES

The ANS consists of two divisions: the sympathetic nervous system and the parasympathetic nervous system. The sympathetic nervous system controls the body's reaction to extreme, stressful, and emergency situations. For example, the sympathetic nervous system increases the heart rate, signals the adrenal glands to secrete adrenaline, triggers the dilation of the pupils, and slows

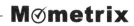

digestion. The parasympathetic nervous system counteracts the effects of the sympathetic nervous system. For example, the parasympathetic nervous system decreases heart rate, signals the adrenal glands to stop secreting adrenaline, constricts the pupils, and returns the digestion process to normal.

> **Review Video: <u>Autonomic Nervous System</u>**
> Visit mometrix.com/academy and enter code: 598501

SOMATIC NERVOUS SYSTEM

The somatic nervous system (SNS) controls the five senses and the voluntary movement of skeletal muscle. So, this system has all of the neurons that are connected to sense organs.

EFFERENT AND AFFERENT NERVES

Efferent (motor) and afferent (sensory) nerves help the somatic nervous system operate the senses and the movement of skeletal muscle. Efferent muscles bring signals from the central nervous system to the sensory organs and the muscles. Afferent muscles bring signals from the sensory organs and the muscles to the central nervous system.

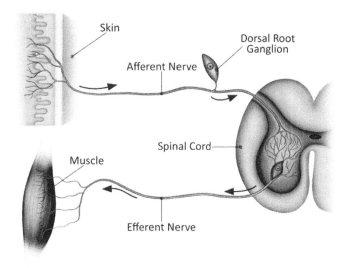

REFLEX ARCS AND REFLEXES

The somatic nervous system also performs involuntary movements which are known as reflex arcs. A reflex, the simplest act of the nervous system, is an automatic response without any conscious thought to a stimulus via the reflex arc. The reflex arc is the simplest nerve pathway, which bypasses the brain and is controlled by the spinal cord. For example, in the classic knee-jerk response (patellar tendon reflex), the stimulus is the reflex hammer hitting the tendon, and the response is the muscle contracting, which jerks the foot upward. The stimulus is detected by sensory receptors, and a message is sent along a sensory (afferent) neuron to one or more interneurons in the spinal cord. The interneuron(s) transmit this message to a motor (efferent) neuron, which carries the message to the correct effector (muscle).

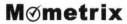

MALE REPRODUCTIVE SYSTEM

The functions of the male reproductive system are to produce, maintain, and transfer **sperm** and **semen** into the female reproductive tract and to produce and secrete **male hormones**.

The external structure includes the penis, scrotum, and testes. The **penis**, which contains the **urethra**, can fill with blood and become erect, enabling the deposition of semen and sperm into the female reproductive tract during sexual intercourse. The **scrotum** is a sack of skin and smooth muscle that houses the testes and keeps the testes outside the body wall at a cooler, proper temperature for **spermatogenesis**. The **testes**, or testicles, are the male gonads, which produce sperm and testosterone.

The internal structure includes the epididymis, vas deferens, ejaculatory ducts, urethra, seminal vesicles, prostate gland, and bulbourethral glands. The **epididymis** stores the sperm as it matures. Mature sperm moves from the epididymis through the **vas deferens** to the **ejaculatory duct**. The **seminal vesicles** secrete alkaline fluids with proteins and mucus into the ejaculatory duct also. The **prostate gland** secretes a milky white fluid with proteins and enzymes as part of the semen. The **bulbourethral**, or Cowper's, glands secrete a fluid into the urethra to neutralize the acidity in the urethra, which would damage sperm.

Additionally, the hormones associated with the male reproductive system include **follicle-stimulating hormone (FSH)**, which stimulates spermatogenesis; **luteinizing hormone (LH)**, which stimulates testosterone production; and **testosterone**, which is responsible for the male sex characteristics. FSH and LH are gonadotropins, which stimulate the gonads (male testes and female ovaries).

HORMONES

The hormones associated with the male reproductive system include:

- follicle-stimulating hormone, which stimulates spermatogenesis
- luteinizing hormone, which stimulates testosterone production
- testosterone, which is responsible for the male sex characteristics

FEMALE REPRODUCTIVE SYSTEM

FUNCTIONS

The functions of the female reproductive system are to produce **ova** (oocytes or egg cells), transfer the ova to the **fallopian tubes** for fertilization, receive the sperm from the male, and provide a protective, nourishing environment for the developing **embryo**.

The external portion of the female reproductive system includes the labia majora, labia minora, Bartholin's glands, and clitoris. The **labia majora** and the **labia minora** enclose and protect the vagina. The **Bartholin's glands** secrete a lubricating fluid. The **clitoris** contains erectile tissue and nerve endings for sensual pleasure.

The internal portion of the female reproductive system includes the ovaries, fallopian tubes, uterus, and vagina. The **ovaries**, which are the female gonads, produce the ova and secrete **estrogen** and **progesterone**. The **fallopian tubes** carry the mature egg toward the uterus. Fertilization typically occurs in the fallopian tubes. If fertilized, the egg travels to the **uterus**, where it implants in the uterine wall. The uterus protects and nourishes the developing embryo until birth. The **vagina** is a

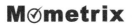

muscular tube that extends from the **cervix** of the uterus to the outside of the body. The vagina receives the semen and sperm during sexual intercourse and provides a birth canal when needed.

Review Video: <u>Reproductive Systems</u>
Visit mometrix.com/academy and enter code: 505450

RESPIRATORY SYSTEM

UPPER AND LOWER RESPIRATORY SYSTEM

The respiratory system can be divided into the upper and lower respiratory system. The **upper respiratory system** includes the nose, nasal cavity, mouth, pharynx, and larynx. The **lower respiratory system** includes the trachea, lungs, and bronchial tree. Alternatively, the components of the respiratory system can be categorized as part of the airway, the lungs, or the respiratory muscles. The **airway** includes the nose, nasal cavity, mouth, pharynx (throat), larynx (voice box), trachea (windpipe), bronchi, and bronchial network. The airway is lined with **cilia** that trap microbes and debris and sweep them back toward the mouth. The **lungs** are structures that house the **bronchi** and bronchial network, which extend into the lungs and terminate in millions of **alveoli** (air sacs). The walls of the alveoli are only one cell thick, allowing for the exchange of gases with the blood capillaries that surround them. The right lung has three lobes. The left lung has only two lobes, leaving room for the heart on the left side of the body. The lungs are surrounded by a **pleural membrane**, which reduces friction between the lungs and walls of the thoracic cavity when breathing. The respiratory muscles include the **diaphragm** and the **intercostal muscles**. The diaphragm is a dome-shaped muscle that separates the thoracic and abdominal cavities; as it contracts, it expands the thoracic cavity which draws air into the lungs. The intercostal muscles are located between the ribs.

ALTERNATIVE TO CATEGORIZING THE RESPIRATORY SYSTEM

Alternatively, the components of the respiratory system can be categorized as part of the airway, the lungs, or the respiratory muscles.

AIRWAY

The airway includes the nose, nasal cavity, mouth, pharynx, (throat), larynx (voice box), trachea (windpipe), bronchi, and bronchial network. The airway is lined with cilia that trap microbes and debris and sweep them back toward the mouth.

CONTENTS OF THE LUNGS

The lungs are structures that house the bronchi and bronchial network, which extend into the lungs and terminate in millions of alveoli (air sacs). The walls of the alveoli are only one cell thick, allowing for the exchange of gases with the blood capillaries that surround them. The right lung has three lobes. The left lung only has two lobes, leaving room for the heart on the left side of the body. The lungs are surrounded by a pleural membrane, which reduces friction between surfaces when breathing.

RESPIRATORY MUSCLES

The features of the respiratory muscles are as follows:

- The respiratory muscles include the diaphragm and the intercostal muscles.
- The diaphragm is a dome-shaped muscle that separates the thoracic and abdominal cavities.
- The intercostal muscles are located between the ribs.

Anatomy and Physiology

FUNCTION

The main function of the respiratory system is to supply the body with **oxygen** and rid the body of **carbon dioxide**. This exchange of gases occurs in millions of tiny **alveoli**, which are surrounded by blood capillaries. The respiratory system also filters air. Air is warmed, moistened, and filtered as it passes through the nasal passages before it reaches the lungs. The respiratory system also allows for speech. As air passes through the throat, it moves through the **larynx** (voice box), which vibrates and produces sound, before it enters the **trachea** (windpipe). Cough production allows foreign particles which have entered the nasal passages or airways to be expelled from the respiratory system. The respiratory system functions in the sense of smell using **chemoreceptors** that are located in the nasal cavity and respond to airborne chemicals. The respiratory system also helps the body maintain acid-base **homeostasis**. Hyperventilation can increase blood pH during **acidosis** (low pH). Slowing breathing during **alkalosis** (high pH) helps lower blood pH.

PRODUCING SPEECH, FILTERING AIR, AND PRODUCING COUGHS

The respiratory system is responsible for speech. As air passes through the throat, it moves through the larynx (voice box), which vibrates and produces sound, before it enters the trachea (windpipe). The respiratory system also filters air. Air is warmed, moistened, and filtered as it passes through the nasal passages before it reaches the lungs. The respiratory system is vital in cough production. Foreign particles entering the nasal passages or airways are expelled from the body by the respiratory system.

SENSE OF SMELL AND MAINTAINING ACID-BASE HOMEOSTASIS

The respiratory system functions in the sense of smell. Chemoreceptors that are located in the nasal cavity respond to airborne chemicals. The respiratory system also helps the body maintain acid-base homeostasis. Hyperventilation can increase blood pH during acidosis (low pH). Slowing breathing during alkalosis (high pH) helps to lower blood pH.

INHALATION AND EXHALATION

During the breathing process, the diaphragm and the intercostal muscles contract to expand the lungs. During inspiration or inhalation, the diaphragm contracts and moves down, increasing the size of the chest cavity. During expiration or exhalation, the intercostal muscles relax and the ribs contract, decreasing the size of the chest cavity. As the volume of the chest cavity increases, the pressure inside the chest cavity decreases. Because the outside air is under a greater amount of pressure than the air inside the lungs, air rushes into the lungs. When the diaphragm and intercostal muscles relax, the size of the chest cavity decreases, forcing air out of the lungs.

MEDULLA OBLONGATA

The breathing process is controlled by the portion of the brain stem called the medulla oblongata. The medulla oblongata monitors the level of carbon dioxide in the blood and signals the breathing rate to increase when these levels are too high.

SKELETAL SYSTEM

The human skeletal system, which consists of 206 bones along with numerous tendons, ligaments, and cartilage, is divided into the axial skeleton and the appendicular skeleton.

The **axial skeleton** consists of 80 bones and includes the vertebral column, rib cage, sternum, skull, and hyoid bone. The **vertebral column** consists of 33 vertebrae classified as cervical vertebrae, thoracic vertebrae, lumbar vertebrae, and sacral vertebrae. The **rib cage** includes 12 paired ribs, 10 pairs of true ribs and two pairs of floating ribs, and the **sternum**, which consists of the manubrium, corpus sterni, and xiphoid process. The **skull** includes the cranium and facial bones. The **ossicles** are bones in the middle ear. The **hyoid bone** provides an attachment point for the tongue muscles. The axial skeleton protects vital organs including the brain, heart, and lungs.

The **appendicular skeleton** consists of 126 bones including the pectoral girdle, pelvic girdle, and appendages. The **pectoral girdle** consists of the scapulae (shoulder blades) and clavicles (collarbones). The **pelvic girdle** attaches to the sacrum at the sacroiliac joint. The upper appendages (arms) include the humerus, radius, ulna, carpals, metacarpals, and phalanges. The lower appendages (legs) include the femur, patella, fibula, tibia, tarsals, metatarsals, and phalanges.

> **Review Video: Skeletal System**
> Visit mometrix.com/academy and enter code: 256447

BASIC FUNCTIONS

The skeletal system serves many functions including providing structural support, providing movement, providing protection, producing blood cells, and storing substances such as fat and minerals. The skeletal system provides the body with structure and support for the muscles and organs.

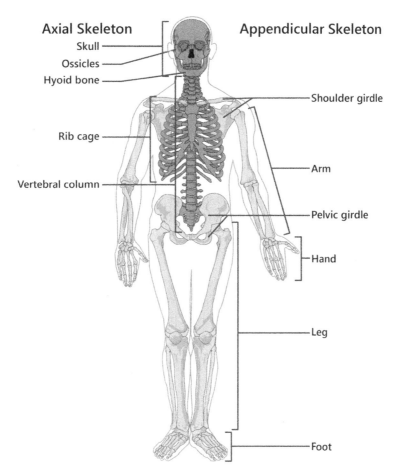

PROVIDING MOVEMENT WITH JOINTS AND THE MUSCULAR SYSTEM

The skeletal system provides movement with joints and the muscular system. Bones provide attachment points for muscles. Joints including hinge joints, ball-and-socket joints, pivot joints, ellipsoid joints, gliding joints, and saddle joints. Each muscle is attached to two bones: the origin

35

and the insertion. The origin remains immobile, and the insertion is the bone that moves as the muscle contracts and relaxes.

PROTECTION OF THE BRAIN, SPINAL CORD, HEART AND LUNGS, AND REPRODUCTIVE ORGANS

The skeletal system serves to protect the body. The cranium protects the brain. The vertebrae protect the spinal cord. The rib cage protects the heart and lungs. The pelvis protects the reproductive organs.

ROLES OF RED MARROW AND YELLOW MARROW

The red marrow manufactures red and white blood cells. All bone marrow is red at birth, but adults have approximately one-half red bone marrow and one-half yellow bone marrow. Yellow bone marrow stores fat.

CALCIUM AND PHOSPHORUS STORAGE

The skeletal system provides a reservoir to store the minerals calcium and phosphorus.

ROLES OF MOVEMENT, MINERAL STORAGE, SUPPORT, PROTECTION, AND BLOOD CELL FORMATION

The skeletal system has an important role in the following body functions:

- **Movement** – The action of skeletal muscles on bones moves the body.
- **Mineral Storage** – Bones serve as storage facilities for essential mineral ions.
- **Support** – Bones act as a framework and support system for the organs.
- **Protection** – Bones surround and protect key organs in the body.
- **Blood Cell Formation** – Red blood cells are produced in the marrow of certain bones.

CLASSIFICATION OF BONES

Bones are classified as long, short, flat, or irregular. Bones are a connective tissue with a base of pulp containing collagen and living cells. Bone tissue is constantly regenerating itself as the mineral composition changes. This allows for special needs during growth periods and maintains calcium levels for the body. Bone regeneration can deteriorate in old age, particularly among women, leading to osteoporosis.

BACKBONE

The flexible and curved backbone is supported by muscles and ligaments. Intervertebral discs are stacked one above another and provide cushioning for the backbone. Trauma or shock may cause these discs to herniate and cause pain. The sensitive spinal cord is enclosed in a cavity which is well protected by the bones of the vertebrae.

ROLE OF JOINTS AND TYPES OF CONNECTIVE BONE TISSUE

Joints are areas of contact adjacent to bones.

- Synovial joints are the most common, and are freely moveable. These may be found at the shoulders and knees.
- Cartilaginous joints fill the spaces between some bones and restrict movement. Examples of cartilaginous joints are those between vertebrae.
- Fibrous joints have fibrous tissue connecting bones and no cavity is present.

Two types of connective bone tissue include compact bone and spongy bone.

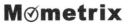

COMPACT BONE AND THE HAVERSIAN SYSTEM

Compact, or cortical, bone, which consists of tightly packed cells, is strong, dense, and rigid. Running vertically throughout compact bone are the Haversian canals, which are surrounded by concentric circles of bone tissue called lamellae. The spaces between the lamellae are called the lacunae. These lamellae and canals along with their associated arteries, veins, lymph vessels, and nerve endings are referred to collectively as the Haversian system. The Haversian system provides a reservoir for calcium and phosphorus for the blood.

SMOOTH, WHITE APPEARANCE OF BONE

Bones have a thin outside layer of compact bone, which gives them their characteristic smooth, white appearance.

SPONGY BONE

Spongy, or cancellous, bone consists of trabeculae, which are a network of girders with open spaces filled with red bone marrow. Compared to compact bone, spongy bone is lightweight and porous, which helps reduce the bone's overall weight.

DIAPHYSIS

In long bones, the diaphysis consists of compact bone surrounding the marrow cavity and spongy bone containing red marrow in the epiphyses.

LIVER

The liver is the largest solid organ of the body. It is also the largest gland. It weighs about three pounds in an adult and is located below the diaphragm on the right side of the abdomen. The liver is made up of four **lobes**: right, left, quadrate, and caudate lobes. The liver is secured to the diaphragm and abdominal walls by five **ligaments**. They are called the falciform (which forms a membrane-like barrier between the right and left lobes), coronary, right triangular, left triangular, and round ligaments.

The liver processes blood once it has received nutrients from the intestines via the **hepatic portal vein**. The **hepatic artery** supplies oxygen-rich blood from the abdominal aorta so that the organ can function. Blood leaves the liver through the **hepatic veins**. The liver's functional units are called **lobules** (made up of layers of liver cells). Blood enters the lobules through branches of the portal vein and hepatic artery. The blood then flows through small channels called **sinusoids**.

VITAL FUNCTIONS IN THE BODY

The liver is responsible for performing many vital functions in the body including:

- Production of bile
- Production of certain blood plasma proteins
- Production of cholesterol (and certain proteins needed to carry fats)
- Storage of excess glucose in the form of glycogen (that can be converted back to glucose when needed)
- Regulation of amino acids
- Processing of hemoglobin (to store iron)
- Conversion of ammonia (that is poisonous to the body) to urea (a waste product excreted in urine)
- Purification of the blood (clears out drugs and other toxins)
- Regulation of blood clotting
- Controlling infections by boosting immune factors and removing bacteria

Anatomy and Physiology

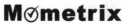

PASSAGE OF NUTRIENTS THROUGH THE LIVER AND ABSORPTION OF NUTRIENTS

The nutrients (and drugs) that pass through the liver are converted into forms that are appropriate for the body to use. In the digestive process, most nutrients are absorbed in the small intestine.

URINARY SYSTEM

The urinary system is capable of eliminating excess substances while preserving the substances needed by the body to function. The urinary system consists of the kidneys, urinary ducts, and bladder.

Review Video: Urinary System
Visit mometrix.com/academy and enter code: 601053

KIDNEYS

The kidneys are bean-shaped organs that are located at the back of the abdominal cavity just under the diaphragm. Each **kidney** (the labelled diagram on the left) consists of the renal cortex (outer layer), renal medulla (inner layer), and renal pelvis, which collects waste products from the nephrons and funnels them to the ureter.

The **renal cortex** (1) is composed of approximately one million **nephrons** (6 and the labelled diagram on the right), which are the tiny, individual filters of the kidneys. Each nephron contains a cluster of capillaries called a **glomerulus** (8) surrounded by the cup-shaped **Bowman's capsule** (9), which leads to a **tubule** (10).

The kidneys receive blood from the **renal arteries (3)**, which branch off the aorta. In general, the kidneys filter the blood (F), reabsorb needed materials (R), and secrete (S) and excrete (E) wastes and excess water in the urine. More specifically, blood flows from the renal arteries into **arterioles** (7) into the glomerulus, where it is filtered. The **glomerular filtrate** enters the **proximal convoluted tubule,** where water, glucose, ions, and other organic molecules are reabsorbed back into the bloodstream through the **renal vein** (4). Reabsorption and secretion occur between the tubules and the **peritubular capillaries** (12).

Additional substances such as urea and drugs are removed from the blood in the **distal convoluted tubule**. Also, the pH of the blood can be adjusted in the distal convoluted tubule by the secretion of **hydrogen ions**. Finally, the unabsorbed materials flow out from the collecting tubules located in the **renal medulla** (2) to the **renal pelvis** as urine. Urine is drained from the kidneys through the

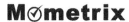

ureters (5) to the **urinary bladder**, where it is stored until expulsion from the body through the **urethra**.

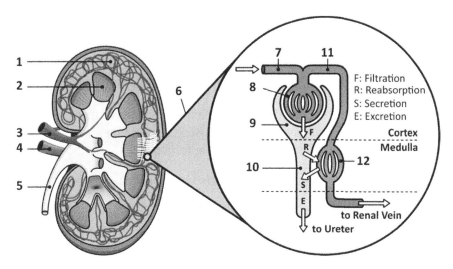

Anatomy and Physiology

Tissue Injury and Repair

IMMUNE SYSTEM

The immune system protects the body against invading **pathogens** including bacteria, viruses, fungi, and protists. The immune system includes the **lymphatic system** (lymph, lymph capillaries, lymph vessel, and lymph nodes) as well as the **red bone marrow** and numerous **leukocytes**, or white blood cells. Tissue fluid enters the **lymph capillaries**, which combine to form **lymph vessels**. Skeletal muscle contractions move the lymph one way through the lymphatic system to lymphatic ducts, which dump back into the venous blood supply and the **lymph nodes**, which are situated along the lymph vessels, and filter the lymph of pathogens and other matter. The lymph nodes are concentrated in the neck, armpits, and groin areas. Outside the lymphatic vessel system lies the **lymphatic tissue,** including the tonsils, adenoids, thymus, spleen, and Peyer's patches. The **tonsils**, located in the pharynx, protect against pathogens entering the body through the mouth and throat. The **thymus** serves as a maturation chamber for immature T cells that are formed in the bone marrow. The **spleen** cleans the blood of dead cells and pathogens. **Peyer's patches**, which are located in the small intestine, protect the digestive system from pathogens.

> **Review Video: Immune System**
> Visit mometrix.com/academy and enter code: 622899

GENERAL IMMUNE DEFENSES

The body's general immune defenses include:

- **Skin** – An intact epidermis and dermis form a formidable barrier against bacteria.
- **Ciliated Mucous Membranes** – Cilia sweep pathogens out of the respiratory tract.
- **Glandular Secretions** – Secretions from exocrine glands destroy bacteria.
- **Gastric Secretions** – Gastric acid destroys pathogens.
- **Normal Bacterial Populations** – Compete with pathogens in the gut and vagina.

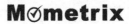

STOPPING INFECTION

Phagocytes and inflammation responses mobilize white blood cells and chemical reactions to stop infection. These responses include localized redness, tissue repair, and fluid-seeping healing agents. Additionally, plasma proteins act as the complement system to repel bacteria and pathogens.

WHITE BLOOD CELLS AND CELLS THAT CONTRIBUTE TO THE BODY'S DEFENSE

Three types of white blood cells form the foundation of the body's immune system. They are:

- **Macrophages** – Phagocytes that alert T cells to the presence of foreign substances.
- **T Lymphocytes** – These directly attack cells infected by viruses and bacteria.
- **B Lymphocytes** – These cells target specific bacteria for destruction.

Memory cells, suppressor T cells, and helper T cells also contribute to the body's defense.

ANTI-BODY MEDIATED AND CELL-MEDIATED IMMUNE RESPONSES

Immune responses can be anti-body mediated when the response is to an antigen, or cell-mediated when the response is to already infected cells. These responses are controlled and measured counter-attacks that recede when the foreign agents are destroyed.

SECONDARY IMMUNE RESPONSE

Once an invader has attacked the body, if it returns it is immediately recognized and a secondary immune response occurs. This secondary response is rapid and powerful, much more so than the original response. These memory lymphocytes circulate throughout the body for years, alert to a possible new attack.

LEUKOCYTES

Leukocytes, or white blood cells, are produced in the red bone marrow. Leukocytes can be classified as monocytes (macrophages and dendritic cells), granulocytes (neutrophils, basophils, and eosinophils), T lymphocytes, B lymphocytes, or natural killer cells.

MONOCYTES AND GRANULOCYTES

Macrophages found traveling in the lymph or fixed in lymphatic tissue are the largest, long-living phagocytes that engulf and destroy pathogens. Dendritic cells present antigens (foreign particles) to T cells. Neutrophils are short-living phagocytes that respond quickly to invaders. Basophils alert the body of invasion. Eosinophils are large, long-living phagocytes that defend against multicellular invaders.

T CELLS AND B CELLS

T lymphocytes or T cells include helper T cells, killer T cells, suppressor T cells, and memory T cells. Helper T cells help the body fight infections by producing antibodies and other chemicals. Killer T cells destroy cells that are infected with a virus or pathogen and tumor cells. Suppressor T cells stop or "suppress" the other T cells when the battle is over. Memory T cells remain in the blood on alert in case the invader attacks again. B lymphocytes, or B cells, produce antibodies.

ANTIGENS

Antigens are substances that stimulate the immune system. Antigens are typically proteins on the surfaces of bacteria, viruses, and fungi. Substances such as drugs, toxins, and foreign particles can also be antigens.

40

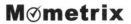

REACTION TO UNFAMILIAR ANTIGENS

The human body recognizes the antigens of its own cells, but it will attack cells or substances with unfamiliar antigens. Specific antibodies are produced for each antigen that enters the body.

TYPICAL IMMUNE RESPONSE

In a typical immune response, when a pathogen or foreign substance enters the body, it is engulfed by a macrophage, which presents fragments of the antigen on its surface. A helper T cell joins the macrophage, and the killer (cytotoxic) T cells and B cells are activated. Killer T cells search out and destroy cells presenting the same antigens. B cells differentiate into plasma cells and memory cells. Plasma cells produce antibodies specific to that pathogen or foreign substance. Antibodies bind to antigens on the surface of pathogens and mark them for destruction by other phagocytes. Memory cells remain in the blood stream to protect against future infections from the same pathogen.

ADAPTIVE IMMUNITY

At birth, an innate immune system protects an individual from pathogens. When an individual encounters infection or has an immunization, the individual develops an adaptive immunity that reacts to pathogens. So, this adaptive immunity is acquired.

NATURALLY AND ARTIFICIALLY ACQUIRED ACTIVE IMMUNITY

A naturally acquired active immunity is natural because the individual is exposed and builds immunity to a pathogen without an immunization. An artificially acquired active immunity is artificial because the individual is exposed and builds immunity to a pathogen by a vaccine.

ARTIFICIALLY ACQUIRED PASSIVE IMMUNITY

An artificially acquired passive immunity is an immunization that is given in recent outbreaks or emergency situations. This immunization provides quick and short-lived protection to disease by the use of antibodies that can come from another person or animal.

Concepts of Energetic Anatomy

QI/CHI

According to Traditional Chinese Medicine (TCM), **qi** or **chi** is the vital force of the universe which flows through the human body in a complex system of energy channels. It is considered the force which gives life the spark, and without it, there would be no action, no movement, and no life. It is believed that these energy channels in which qi/chi flows can be manipulated and palpated using massage or needles, as in acupuncture. It is the basis of TCM that disturbances in this flow of energy are what cause disease and dysfunction. If the energy system is in balance and flowing freely, then there is the presence of health and well-being. When the qi/chi flow is strong, the person will have more life force, which means they will be more alert, active, and present. In the absence of qi/chi, the person will be sluggish and feel fatigued. Acupuncture and massage can increase the flow of qi/chi.

YIN AND YANG

Yin and yang is the concept on which the system of Traditional Chinese Medicine (TCM) is based. It is the concept that there is a polarity to the universe, a balance that is ever-changing. Yin refers to the shady side of a hill, while yang is the sunny side. Anything that is dark, heavy, or slow is yin and things that are bright, active, or fast are yang. Yin and yang are not meant to restrictively define something, but instead are relative. There is a relationship between the two parts of anything. Water can become a gas, which is fine and free; or it can become ice, which is hard and cold. Each

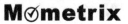

cannot exist without the other. They are the polar opposites of each other. They each serve to keep the other in check and there must be a constant balancing and rebalancing. When yin and yang are in balance, there is well-being.

THEORY OF THE FIVE ELEMENTS

The theory of the Five Elements breaks down our existence into five fundamental energies, substances, and qualities. The Five Elements are wood, fire, earth, metal, and water. Each element has correspondences, both in the body and in nature, and its own energy channel. The elements interact with each other. Each element controls and is controlled by another element. When one element is especially strong, it can either control or nourish another element. An element that is too weak can fail to nourish or it can be easily overcome by another element. The elements correspond to different organs in the body as well as emotions. When an element is too weak or too strong, it can manifest as a dysfunction in an organ or an increase or decrease in a particular emotion. The Five Elements are used as a diagnostic tool in Asian bodywork therapies. The goal is to balance the cyclic relationship among the elements in order to foster the healthiest life.

SEVEN CHAKRAS

The body is said to contain seven **chakras** that descend along the midline of the body starting at the crown of the skull and ending just above the pelvic bone. These focal areas, typically depicted as vortices, serve as conduits for distributing and reabsorbing the body's energy. They are often described as being open, aligned, or in balance (when working properly), or as being blocked, misaligned, or out of balance (when not working properly). Each chakra embodies a specific trait or spiritual concern.

Chakra Name	Chakra Location	Main Concern
Crown	Top of head	Spirituality
Third Eye	Above and between eyebrows	Intuition, wisdom
Throat	Base of neck	Communication, self-expression
Heart	Chest at heart	Love and relationships
Solar Plexus	Above navel	Personal power, self will
Sacral	Below navel	Emotional balance, sexuality
Root	Pelvic floor	Survival, physical needs

POLARITY THERAPY

Polarity therapy, developed by Randolph Stone in the mid-1900s, is a complex form of therapy using the concepts of energy and the body's innate capacity for health. Through his studies of ancient healing traditions, Stone discovered the common belief that there is a subtle form of life energy that flows through the body and gives it health, and that the obstruction of this flow of energy is the cause of disease. His teachings are eclectic and hard to define, but pull from great traditions such as traditional Chinese medicine, acupuncture, Ayurvedic medicine, and herbal medicine. Most polarity therapists use it as a framework for their sessions. There are many different techniques the practitioner can use and develop their own techniques based on his teachings. The goal of a session is to unblock the life energy. This is done by affecting muscular relaxation, balancing the autonomic nervous system, and creating structural change. The techniques used are a variety of hand positions that involve cradling, rocking, and pulling in specific ways to stimulate the flow of blocked energy in the body.

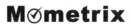

THERAPEUTIC TOUCH

Therapeutic touch is commonly used by nurses and is a simpler form of energy therapy. It can be used by anyone without formal training and is a form of compassionate healing. The teachings of therapeutic touch are that each person is ingrained with a natural ability to heal and that we can be a vessel for healing without having had any specialized training or education. Even though the technique is called therapeutic touch, it actually requires no physical touch. The hands are held above and off the body and are used to adjust the aura or human energy field. During a session, the practitioner will hold their hands 2-6 inches over the skin and move them over the body in sweeping motions, as if smoothing out wrinkles in the patient's energy field. The therapy should facilitate a feeling of relaxation and well-being. It has been shown to reduce the signs of tension and stimulate the body's immune response. It is often used to decrease the effects of chemotherapy and radiation.

MERIDIANS

The concept of a system of energy channels in the body, known as meridians, can be traced back to ancient China. The Chinese developed this system as a way to describe the anatomy and physiology of the body through observation. Each meridian or channel corresponds to an organ of the body. The meridians lined through the body do not necessarily correspond to the location of the organ. Meridians exist in corresponding pairs and can be considered the body's energy highways. Each meridian has multiple acupuncture points along its path. There are 12 main meridians and each limb has six that travel it. There is a specific pattern in which the energy flows, starting with the chest and down the arms, then back up the arms to the neck and head before flowing down the body through the legs to the feet and back up to the chest to start the pattern again.

PURPOSE OF MOST ENERGY THERAPIES

Energetic healing arts have been practiced by many cultures in history. Each has their own name for the energy or life force that flows through the body. Most of the energetic healing arts being practiced today come from the studies of healing in China and India, with China being the most prevalent. The purpose of these therapies has been to treat disruptions in the flow of energy throughout the body that are seen as the cause of disease and dysfunction. It is believed that, when the flow of energy is strong and allowed to move freely through the body, there will be an abundance of energy, health, and well-being. When the energy is blocked, the body is not able to exist at its highest potential and it suffers from fatigue and sluggishness and organs become diseased. Energy therapies serve to prevent and heal this dysfunction in the energy flow.

PHYSIOLOGICAL EFFECTS OF ENERGETIC MANIPULATION

Energetic manipulation has been shown to be effective in treating a broad range of conditions. The goal of energetic manipulation is to bring the body's energy flow back into balance. The most common physiological effects that are seen with the manipulation of energy are a decrease in blood pressure, a sense of calm or relaxation, better sleep at night, and a strengthening of the immune system. Clients also report a feeling of calm, decreased joint pain, increased mobility, and greater range of motion. There can at times be negative effects from energetic manipulation. These negative effects are generally limited to dizziness, headache, or anxiety. Some people with mental health disorders such as schizophrenia or bipolar disorders may have negative reactions, but most energetic manipulation techniques are considered safe for all populations.

REFLEXOLOGY WORK

The concept of reflexology is that, by applying pressure to certain points, the practitioner can stimulate benefits in distant areas of the body that correspond to that point. These are links that are

Anatomy and Physiology

43

activated by stimulating reflex points which relieve tension, improve blood supply, and normalize bodily functions. The practitioner finds these points by feeling for areas of swelling, knots, or crunchiness in the tissue. These changes occur due to a reflex arc. The brain sends signals to a reflex point corresponding to an organ that is in distress and has become inflamed and congested. When the practitioner finds this point and stimulates it, the signal returns to the brain, which then sends endorphins to the impacted area, increasing blood flow and lowering the inflammation and distress. All of these reflex points can be found on the hands and the feet and there is a standard map of points which can be worked by the practitioner.

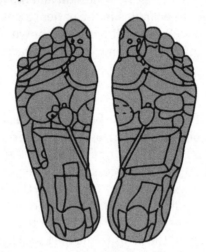

Kinesiology

Components and Characteristics of Muscles

TRAITS OF THE THREE TYPES OF MUSCLE TISSUE

- Skeletal muscle tissue:
  - Voluntary – under conscious control
  - Responsible for movement
  - Attached to bone or other muscles by tendons
  - Striated – light and dark cross-markings
- Smooth Muscle Tissue
  - Involuntary – controlled by involuntary nerve impulses from the autonomic nervous system or glandular activity
  - Responsible for movement of food through the digestive tract, the constriction of blood vessels, and the emptying of the bladder
  - Found in the hollow organs of the stomach, small intestine, colon, bladder, and blood vessels
  - Non-striated
- Cardiac Muscle Tissue
  - Occurs only in the heart
  - Involuntary
  - Responsible for the beating of the heart and pumps blood through the heart and into the blood vessels
  - Contains cell junctions called intercalated discs

CHARACTERISTICS THAT ENABLE MUSCLES TO PERFORM THEIR FUNCTIONS

There are four identified characteristics of muscles that allow them to function as intended:

- **Irritability**: Irritability refers to a muscle's ability to be stimulated to action, whether by internal means such as a nerve impulse or by external means such as pressure, heat, or electrical current. This characteristic may also be referred to as **excitability**.
- **Contractility**: Contractility refers to a muscle's ability to contract. When a muscle contracts, it generates force, pressure, motion, or some combination of these. For example, the muscles of the heart contract to pressurize and pump the blood throughout the body, while the skeletal muscles work in tandem to produce the motion of the body's frame.
- **Extensibility** and **elasticity**: The last two characteristics of muscles are closely related. Extensibility refers to a muscle's ability to stretch and deform without being damaged, while elasticity refers to a muscle's ability to return to its original shape and size after being stretched. These are obviously very important since muscles are expanding and contracting all the time.

ENDOMYSIUM, EPIMYSIUM, AND PERIMYSIUM

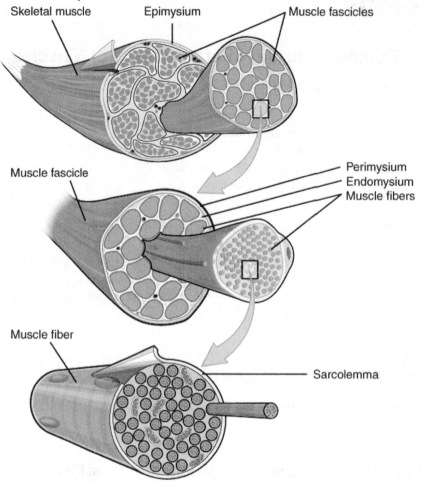

The endomysium, epimysium, and perimysium are layers of fascia that serve to separate the muscular system into compartments and allow it to work properly. These layers of fascia serve as an organizer and compartmentalize the muscles into functional groups:

- **Epimysium** is the most superficial of the fascial layers. It covers each individual muscle in the muscular system.
- **Perimysium** is the middle layer of fascia. It extends inward from the epimysium and separates the muscle into bundles of muscle fibers called fascicles.
- **Endomysium** is the innermost layer of fascia. This layer covers each individual muscle fiber. All three of these layers are vitally important to the function of the muscle. Muscle tissue and fascia work together functionally and structurally to organize and connect muscle to tendons and tendons to bones. This structure is what allows the muscular system to create movement.

COMPONENTS OF MUSCLE FIBER

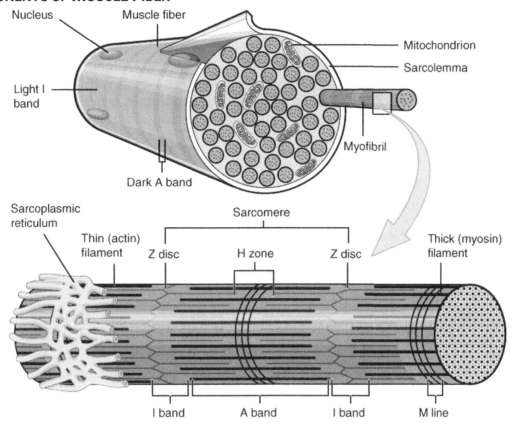

The basic components of a muscle fiber are as follows:

- **Sarcolemma** - The muscle fiber's plasma membrane which is located just beneath the layer of connective tissue covering the muscle fiber.
- **Myofibrils** – The small threadlike structures which are the contractile elements of the muscle. They extend the entire length of the muscle fiber and are striated.
- **Sarcomere** – This is the basic functional unit of the myofibril, where the actin and myosin are contained.
- **Actin** – One of the contractile proteins of a muscle. Actin is associated with thin filaments and interacts with myosin during a muscle contraction.
- **Myosin** – One of the contractile proteins of a muscle. Myosin is associated with thick filaments and interacts with actin during a muscle contraction.
- **A Band** – The A band is located in the middle of the sarcomere. It is caused by myosin filaments.
- **M Line** – The M line is the midline of the sarcomere.
- **H Zone** – This is the zone where the myosin filament is not overlapped by the actin filament.
- **I Band** – This band contains only the actin filaments.
- **Zone of Overlap** – This zone contains both actin and myosin and is where the contraction takes place.
- **Z Line** – The Z line is anchor of the actin filaments and the boundary between sarcomeres.

Kinesiology

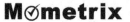

Concepts of Muscle Contractions

SLIDING FILAMENT THEORY OF MUSCLE CONTRACTION

Muscle contraction occurs when the heads of the myosin filaments attach to the thin filaments and begin pulling them toward the M line. The thin filaments then will meet at the center of a sarcomere. This causes the sarcomere to shorten, but the lengths of the myosin and actin filaments do not change. When the sarcomeres shorten, the muscle fiber shortens, which will then cause the shortening of the entire muscle. In this process, the zone of overlap will become larger, the I line becomes narrower, and the Z lines will move closer together. This process requires a constant supply of ATP.

PRIME MOVER, ANTAGONIST, AGONIST, SYNERGIST, AND FIXATOR IN A MUSCLE GROUP

The prime mover, antagonist, agonist, synergist, and fixator in a muscle group are explained below:

- **The prime mover** is the muscle responsible for a specific movement.
- The **agonist** is the muscle that is the prime mover.
- The **antagonist** is the muscle which performs the movement which is the direct opposite of the movement of the agonist.
- **Synergists** are muscles that assist the agonist it its movements.
- **Fixators** are muscles that stabilize more proximal parts so that the distal parts can perform movements.

In order for the body to create movement at a joint, there must be an interaction of a variety of muscles. The prime mover or agonist will contract to create the movement while the antagonist will simultaneously perform the opposite movement in order to allow the primary movement to occur. At the same time, synergists will provide assistance to the primary movement to create more force and stability. The fixator muscles will prevent any movement that would detract from the primary movement and cause a lack of stability.

PRODUCTION OF ATP

ATP (adenosine triphosphate) is an enzyme which is the source of energy for muscular contractions. When the muscle contracts, it causes a release of one of the phosphates in ATP, forming ADP (adenosine diphosphate). In order to re-bond the phosphate, another enzyme, creatine phosphate, will release energy when it contacts ADP and produce ATP. This happens within a fraction of a second. This contraction can only be sustained for a few seconds, however, due to the fact that there is not a sufficient amount of ATP and creatine phosphate in the muscle cell. The other way the cells produce ATP from ADP is through the use of cellular respiration. Both aerobic (using oxygen) and anaerobic respiration convert ADP to ATP, but anaerobic respiration, being less sustainable, is only used when the cell doesn't have sufficient oxygen.

ISOTONIC AND ISOMETRIC MUSCULAR CONTRACTIONS

Isotonic and isometric are forms of muscular contraction. When a muscle contracts, it generates tension, or the force of contraction. This tension is what pulls the two muscle attachment points closer together. When the tension or force generated by the muscle is greater than the resistance of the object being moved, the muscle will shorten and movement will occur. This is an isotonic contraction. If the muscular force is not greater than the resistance, then the muscle will not shorten and no movement will occur. This is an isometric contraction. An example of an isometric contraction would be holding a book in your outstretched hand. The force of resistance of the book is equal to the tension created in the hand. There will be no movement. If the book is raised and lifted, then that would be an isotonic contraction.

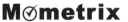

ECCENTRIC VS. CONCENTRIC MUSCULAR CONTRACTION

Eccentric and concentric muscular contractions are the two types of isotonic contractions. This means there is movement happening during the contraction. During a concentric contraction, the muscle is shortening and pulling on another structure such as a tendon. This produces movement and brings the two ends of the muscle closer together, reducing the angle of the joint. In an eccentric contraction, the muscle length is increasing and its ends are getting farther apart, which increases the angle of the joint. An example of a concentric contraction would be picking up a book, while lowering it back down would be the eccentric contraction.

MUSCLE SPINDLES

Muscle spindle cells are specialized cells that have both sensory and motor functions. These cells are interspersed among regular skeletal muscle cells and are found mainly in the belly of the muscle. They are made up of specialized contractile tissue called intrafusal muscle fibers. They are important to the control and coordination of the muscle. Muscle spindle cells function in proprioception, which is the body's ability to recognize its position in space. Muscle spindles monitor changes in the length of the skeletal muscle and how far and fast it is moving and report that information back to the central nervous system. This assists in the coordination of muscle contractions. Muscle spindle cells also report if the muscle is being overstretched and activate a reflex that will prevent injury by stopping the overstretching of the muscle.

SKELETAL MUSCLE TISSUE

Skeletal muscle tissue is composed of fibrous tissue arranged in bundles called fascicles. These fascicles are made up of muscle fibers connected to one another through connective tissue. An extensive supply of blood and lymph vessels, capillaries, and nerve fibers are contained within skeletal muscle tissue. The muscle receives its supply of oxygen through the blood vessels. There are two types of skeletal muscle fibers: type I and type II. Type I muscle fibers are characterized by a large number of reddish fibers, which provide excellent endurance for the muscle through oxidative metabolism. Type II fibers are white in color, and are more suitable for shorter bursts of energy or when speed is required. They rely on anaerobic metabolism for energy and tire more easily. The composition of an individual's skeletal muscle tissue is determined by genetics and by the type of exercise they do on a regular basis.

MUSCLE SHAPES

The muscles of the human body can be numerous shapes, depending on their function. In the trapezius, for instance, the muscle fibers are arranged in a broad, flat pattern, and attach at a large number of points along the scapula. The bicep, on the other hand, is a long, narrow muscle. The muscles of the deep back are very short, and appear as knotty bundles along the spinal column. Longer muscles are generally capable of producing highly visible external movements, and are used to transport heavy objects, for example. Small, deep muscles are usually responsible for precise, balancing adjustments. Muscles that only cross over one joint are called monoarticular, while those that extend across and move more than one joint are called polyarticular.

TENDON ORGANS

Tendon organs are sensory nerve endings located in the area known as the musculotendinous junction. This is where muscle fibers attach to tendons. Their purpose is to measure the tension produced in the muscle cells due to contraction and relaxation and the force pulling on the bone where the tendon attaches. This information is sent to the central nervous system, which is then able to activate tendon reflexes, causing muscle relaxation if the muscle force becomes too strong. This will prevent injury to the muscle, tendon, and the bone to which the tendon is attached.

Kinesiology

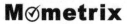

CHARACTERISTICS OF MUSCLES RELATED TO THEIR MOVEMENT

Muscles are able to perform their various functions because they possess certain characteristics. These characteristics are described using the following terms: irritability, contractility, elasticity and extensibility. Irritability refers to the ability of muscles to receive and react to stimuli from outside the body, such as the touch of massage, or to respond to internal stimuli, such as electrical currents sent from the brain. The muscle's irritability also refers to their reaction to heat, chemicals such as acids or salts, and other impulses. Contractility refers to muscles that are capable of shortening and therefore exerting force. An example of a muscle that possesses contractility the cardiac muscle, which forces blood through the body as a result of the pumping action of the heart. Elasticity refers to the ability of a muscle to return to its original shape after being stretched. Extensibility is the ability of muscle to stretch beyond its original shape.

Proprioceptors

PROPRIOCEPTION

Proprioception is the body's ability to recognize its position in space. Even with your eyes closed, you can identify where your arm is in relation to your torso. This happens due to the constant influx of messages received from proprioceptors. These messages inform us of such things as which muscles are being contracted, the positions of the joints, and the level of tension in the tendons. These proprioceptive sensations allow us to walk, eat, and brush our teeth without using our eyes. The brain is continually receiving these messages and making adjustments, which ensure coordination and balance. Proprioceptors are located throughout the body and monitor sensations. Muscle spindles, for example, send messages regarding skeletal muscle length, and Golgi tendon organs monitor the force of a skeletal muscle contraction. Both of these play an important role in movement and muscular effort. Hair cells of the inner ear are also proprioceptors. They provide information critical to maintaining balance and equilibrium. Joint kinesthetic receptors also play an important role in proprioception. These receptors are found within and around the joint capsules of synovial joints. They are responsible for sending sensory signals regarding pressure and acceleration and deceleration of joints.

Locations, Attachments, Actions and Fiber Directions of Muscles

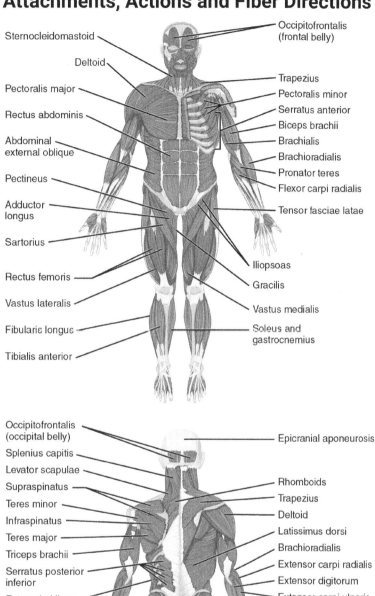

Sternocleidomastoid
Deltoid
Pectoralis major
Rectus abdominis
Abdominal external oblique
Pectineus
Adductor longus
Sartorius
Rectus femoris
Vastus lateralis
Fibularis longus
Tibialis anterior

Occipitofrontalis (frontal belly)
Trapezius
Pectoralis minor
Serratus anterior
Biceps brachii
Brachialis
Brachioradialis
Pronator teres
Flexor carpi radialis
Tensor fasciae latae
Iliopsoas
Gracilis
Vastus medialis
Soleus and gastrocnemius

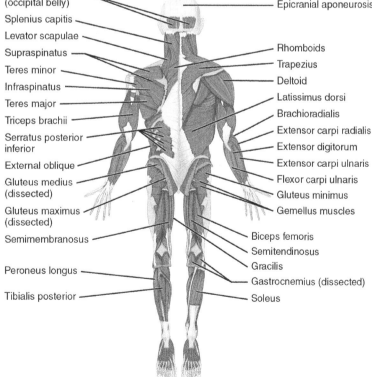

Occipitofrontalis (occipital belly)
Splenius capitis
Levator scapulae
Supraspinatus
Teres minor
Infraspinatus
Teres major
Triceps brachii
Serratus posterior inferior
External oblique
Gluteus medius (dissected)
Gluteus maximus (dissected)
Semimembranosus
Peroneus longus
Tibialis posterior

Epicranial aponeurosis
Rhomboids
Trapezius
Deltoid
Latissimus dorsi
Brachioradialis
Extensor carpi radialis
Extensor digitorum
Extensor carpi ulnaris
Flexor carpi ulnaris
Gluteus minimus
Gemellus muscles
Biceps femoris
Semitendinosus
Gracilis
Gastrocnemius (dissected)
Soleus

Kinesiology

51

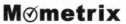

RELATIONSHIP BETWEEN THE MUSCLES AND THE SKELETON

Muscles help to support the framework of the skeletal system. They assist with the movement of the body. Skeletal muscles are those which are striated and attached to the bones through tendons. When muscles constrict or expand, they exert a force on the tendon. The tendon pushes or pulls the bone, which causes the limb or appendage to move. Tendons are not as elastic as muscles, so the majority of the body's movement is due to muscles. Skeletal muscles are primarily voluntary. They do, however, possess some involuntary characteristics that can also cause the muscle to contract or expand. Massage focuses on a therapeutic regimen designed to enhance the function of muscles through techniques that bring about relaxation, release of toxins, greater flexibility, and a greater range of motion. All of these results are accomplished through specific, pressurized body movements.

POINT OF INSERTION

Muscles are connected by tendons that extend from either end of the muscle. In order for movement to occur, one side of the muscle, generally the part closest to the center of the body, is considered the point of origin. This area is not as flexible as the other end of the muscle because of the lack of space in the area, and also because a broader range of motion is not necessary in that area. At the other end of the muscle lies the insertion point. This area is more distal, and the majority of the movement takes place here. Both the origin and the insertion point of the muscle are attached to the bone by a tendon. When one knows the origin of the muscle, it is easy to infer which way the muscle will contract based on that knowledge.

PRIME MOVER AND ANTAGONIST MOVEMENTS OF MUSCLES

Although muscles are distinct within the body, they work in conjunction with other muscles to perform actions. As such, the muscle performing the primary movement is known as the prime mover, or the agonist. To counteract this initial movement, a muscle on the opposite side causes an opposite reaction. This muscle is known as the antagonist. For example, a bicep that contracts would be the agonist, while a triceps that expands would be classified as the antagonist. It is important to understand the relationship between the muscles so an appropriate treatment plan that takes the movement of both muscles into consideration can be created. Any muscles that assist the prime mover are called synergists. A fixator is any muscle that helps to stabilize a body part so another muscle can move.

MOVEMENT OF THE SCAPULA

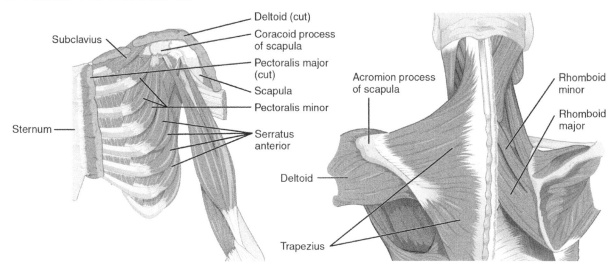

Pectoral girdle muscle (left anterior lateral view)   Pectoral girdle muscles (posterior view)

TRAPEZIUS MUSCLE

The scapula is located on the posterior upper region of the body, and connects the arm bone to the collarbone. The scapula is also known as the shoulder blade, while the collarbone is referred to as the clavicle. The trapezius muscle is connected to the cervical spine from the occipital bone at the top of the spine down to the T5-T12 area of the lumbar column. Three types of trapezius muscles exist: upper, middle, and lower. Each corresponds to the region in which the muscles originate. These muscles are involved with the elevation, depression, and upward rotation of the scapula.

RHOMBOID MUSCLE

There are major and minor components of the rhomboid muscle. The rhomboid major can be found in the T2-T5 portion of the thoracic vertebral column. It is located deep within the trapezius muscle. The purpose of the rhomboid major is to keep the scapula in line with the ribcage. This muscle functions by pulling the scapula closer to the vertebral column. The rhomboid minor retracts the scapula downward. It is found between the C7-T1 vertebral column. Its point of insertion is at the base of the scapula.

LEVATOR SCAPULAE, PECTORALIS MINOR, AND SERRATUS ANTERIOR

The levator scapulae originates from the C1-4 vertebral column, which is located at the back and side of the neck. It helps to move the neck from side to side laterally. It inserts at the top third of the scapula. The pectoralis minor originates between the 3rd and 5th ribs, close to the costal cartilage. The pectoralis minor draws the scapula downward and towards the thorax. It attaches on the coracoid process, which extends outward from the scapula. The serratus anterior originates from anterior ribs 1-8 and causes an upward movement of the scapula. It provides stabilization and is also referred to as the "boxer's muscle" because it assists with protraction of the scapula.

Kinesiology

ARM MUSCLES

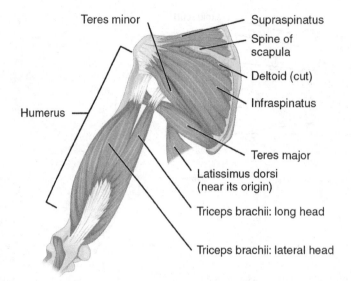

Approximately eight separate muscles cause the upper arm to move. These muscles are listed below:

- **Pectoralis Major** (Clavicular and Sternal) – helps to push the shoulder forward and rotate the arm towards the body
- **Coracobrachialis** – helps the arm swing forward
- **Deltoid** (Anterior, Middle, and Posterior) – mainly responsible for lifting the arm away from the trunk at the shoulder
- **Supraspinatus** – primarily involved in abduction of the shoulder
- **Infraspinatus** – helps to extend the arm and rotate it to the outside
- **Subscapularis** – involved in the medial rotation of the arm
- **Teres minor** – involved with the adduction and lateral rotation of the arm
- **Teres major** – involved with arm extension and medial rotation
- **Latissimus Dorsi** – the major muscle of the upper back, which assists in moving the arm backward and rotating it inward

PECTORALIS MAJOR AND CORACOBRACHIALIS

The pectoralis major is divided into two groups: the clavicular portion and the sternal portion. The clavicular portion originates medially at the clavicle and inserts at the outer ridge of the bicipital groove. Its causative actions are the conduction of adduction, the moving of the limb closer to the body, medial rotation, and flexion of the humerus bone. The humerus is the long bone extending from the scapula at the shoulder to the radius and ulna at the elbow. The sternal portion of the pectoralis major originates from the sternum and the costal cartilage of ribs 1-6, but inserts at the outer ridge of the bicipital groove proximally. It acts on the arm in the same manner and also causes the extension of the humerus when it is flexed. The coracobrachialis originates at the coracoid process of the scapula (the portion of the scapula that extends frontward), and inserts at the middle of the humerus. It assists with the flexion and adduction of the humerus bone.

DELTOID MUSCLE

The deltoid is a triangular-shaped muscle that provides the rounded shape to the human shoulder. It is divided into three sections: anterior, middle, and posterior. The main motion associated with the deltoid is the abduction of the arm. The anterior section originates at the outside third of the

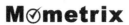

clavicle. It inserts at the deltoid tuberosity of the humerus, and causes flexion and horizontal rotation of the humerus. The middle deltoid muscle originates at the acromion process of the scapula, and also inserts at the deltoid tuberosity. It assists with the abduction of the humerus to a 90-degree extension. The posterior deltoid originates at the lower part of the scapula and inserts at the deltoid tuberosity. It causes the extension, horizontal abduction, and lateral rotation of the humerus.

SUPRASPINATUS, INFRASPINATUS, AND SUBSCAPULARIS

The supraspinatus muscle originates at the supraspinous fossa of the scapula at the superior portion of this bone. Its insertion point is at the top of the humerus bone. This muscle acts upon the upper arm by instigating abduction in the humerus. The infraspinatus muscle originates at the infraspinous fossa of the scapula at the medial portion of this bone. It covers a much larger surface area than the supraspinous fossa. This muscle inserts at the greater tubercle, or large round nodule, of the humerus and assists in the lateral rotation of the humerus. The subscapularis muscle originates at the back surface of the scapula. This muscle inserts at the lesser tubercle of the humerus. Its function is to assist in the medial rotation of the humerus.

TERES MAJOR, TERES MINOR, AND LATISSIMUS DORSI

The teres major is a thick, flat muscle located on the dorsal inferior side of the scapula. The insertion point is the lesser tubercle of the humerus. This muscle extends upward into the tubercle and is responsible for moving the humerus in a way that causes the arm to lower and move in a backward motion. The teres minor is a narrow, long muscle that is part of the rotator cuff. The insertion point is the lowest end of the greater tubercle of the humerus. It causes the humerus to move in a backward motion and also to rotate outward. The latissimus dorsi is a large, triangular, flat muscle located on the posterior side of the body. It covers the lumbar region and the last six of the thoracic vertebrae. This muscle extends upwards to insert at the intertubercular groove of the humerus. The actions it is responsible for are the extension, adduction, and internal rotation of the joint at the shoulder.

BICEPS BRACHII

The biceps brachii is the muscle located on the anterior upper arm. It is often referred to simply as the bicep. Its main purpose is to cause the flexion of the arm. The origin of the bicep is at the coracoid process of the scapula (short head) and the glenoid fossa (long head). It then extends down the arm and attaches at the radial tuberosity, a large nodule at the end of the radius. Because of the insertion point, the biceps brachii also influences the movement of the forearm. There are three actions caused by the biceps brachii: flexion of the forearm, extension of the arm above the shoulder joint, and the supination of the forearm (forearm rotation that results in the palms facing upwards). The triceps brachii is located on the posterior region of the upper arm. It originates at three points: the infraglenoid tuberosity of the scapula, the proximal half of the humerus, and the distal region of the humerus. The triceps brachii is responsible for extending the elbow. The biceps and triceps work in conjunction as flexors and extensors. The flexor contracts the muscle, causing the joint to bend, while the contraction of the extensor causes the limb to return to its original position.

SUPINATOR MUSCLE, PRONATOR TERES, AND PRONATOR QUADRATUS

The supinator is a wide muscle that curves around the upper third of the radius. Its main purpose is to allow the hand and forearm to supinate, or twist, so that the palm of the hand either faces the body or faces forward. It also uses the bicep brachii muscle to perform this action. The supinator consists of two types of fibers: the superficial fibers and the upper fibers. This muscle can be difficult to palpate. The pronator teres and the pronator quadratus are two muscles that work together to pronate the hand so that the palm faces downwards towards the floor. The pronator teres originates at both the humerus and the ulna. It then attaches at the radius. The pronator quadratus runs from the distal part of the anterior ulna to the distal part of the anterior radius. This muscle assists not only with moving the palm to face downwards, but also with keeping the bones of the radius and ulna together.

FLEXION OF THE WRIST

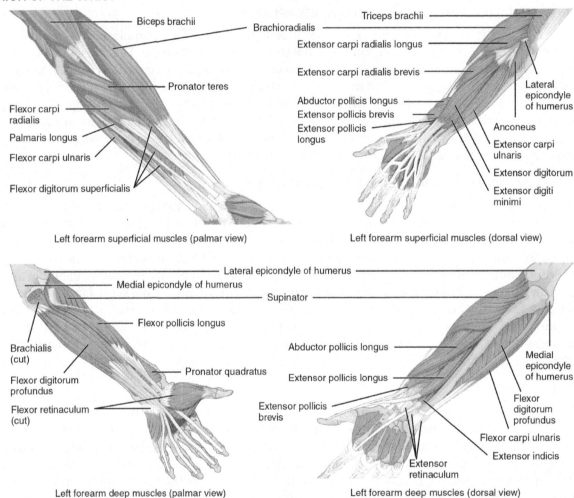

Left forearm superficial muscles (palmar view)

Left forearm superficial muscles (dorsal view)

Left forearm deep muscles (palmar view)

Left forearm deep muscles (dorsal view)

The muscles that play a part in causing flexion of the wrist are:

- **Flexor Carpal Radialis** – This muscle can be felt on the anterior side of the forearm. It can be palpated on the radial side of the palmaris longus tendon; it helps to flex and adduct the hand.
- **Flexor Carpal Ulnaris** (humeral head and ulnar head) – This muscle is located on the proximal half of the forearm; it helps to flex and adduct the hand.
- **Palmaris Longus** – This muscle originates from the humerus and inserts at the palmar aponeurosis, also known as the muscles of the palm of the hand. Somewhat superfluous, this muscle assumes a more prominent role when other muscles are injured.

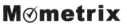

EXTENSION OF THE WRIST

The muscles that play a role in causing the extension of the wrist are:

- **Extensor Carpi Radialis Longus** – This muscle originates at the distal third of the humerus and inserts at the base of 2nd metacarpal or index finger. It moves the wrist in such a way that the hand is moved away from the palm and towards the thumb.
- **Extensor Carpi Radialis Brevis** – This muscle originates on the lateral side of the humerus and inserts at the base of the 3rd metacarpal, or middle finger. It holds the wrist in place during flexion of the fingers and aids in the adduction of the hand.
- **Extensor Carpi Ulnaris** – This muscle originates on the lateral humerus and inserts at the lateral base of the 5th metacarpal, or pinky finger; it extends and adducts the wrist.

MUSCLES THAT ACT UPON THE FINGERS

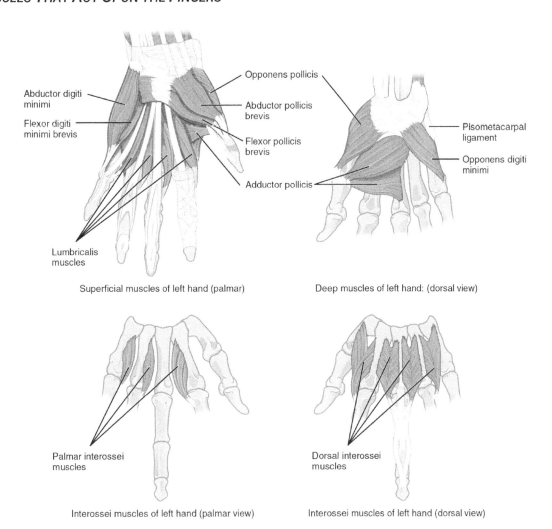

Superficial muscles of left hand (palmar)

Deep muscles of left hand: (dorsal view)

Interossei muscles of left hand (palmar view)

Interossei muscles of left hand (dorsal view)

The following is a list of the muscles that act upon the fingers:

- **Flexor Digitorum Superficialis** – (includes humeral head, ulnar head, and radial and head); flexes the wrist, interphalangeal joints, and hand
- **Flexor Digitorum Profundus** – flexes the distal and proximal interphalangeal joints, metacarpophalangeal joints (except the thumb), and the hand

57

- **Flexor Digiti Minimi** – flexes the little finger
- **Extensor Digitorum** – extends the wrist and the fingers (except the thumb)
- **Extensor Indicis** – extends the metacarpophalangeal joint of the index finger
- **Extensor Digiti Minimi** – helps to extend the wrist and the fifth metacarpophalangeal joint
- **Abductor Digiti Minimi** – abducts and flexes the fifth metacarpophalangeal joint
- **Opponens Digiti Minimi** – coordinates the movements of the little finger in relation to the thumb
- **Palmar Interosseous** – (includes first, second, third, and fourth); helps to flex and adduct the metacarpophalangeal joints
- **Dorsal Interosseous** – adducts the 2nd and 4th metacarpophalangeal joints, assists in radial and ulnar deviation of the 3rd metacarpophalangeal joint, and flexes the 2nd, 3rd, and 4th metacarpophalangeal joints
- **Lumbricals** – flexes the metacarpophalangeal joints and extends the interphalangeal joints

Leg Muscles

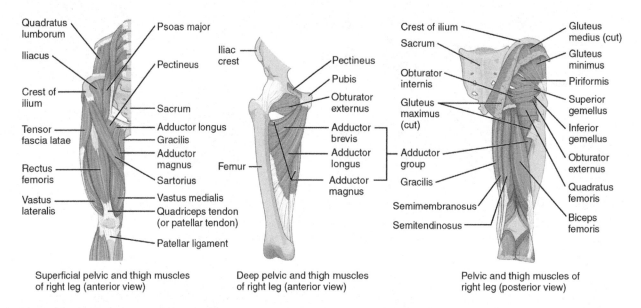

Superficial pelvic and thigh muscles of right leg (anterior view)

Deep pelvic and thigh muscles of right leg (anterior view)

Pelvic and thigh muscles of right leg (posterior view)

Larger Muscles That Act Upon the Thigh and the Lateral Rotators

The muscles of the lateral rotators and thigh are made up of the gluteus maximus, which provides for lateral movement and support of the thigh, the gluteus medius, which adducts the thigh, and the gluteus minimus, which assists with rotating the hip. The internal rotators include the quadratus femoris, the obturator externus and internus, and the gemellus superior and inferior. These muscles aid in rotating the hip area. Additional muscle groups include the adductor brevis, the adductor longus, and the adductor magnus. These muscles assist with the extension and rotation of the thigh. The psoas major and the iliacus are located in the pelvic region, and assist with flexing the thigh and hip and rotating the knee.

Muscles That Act on the Upper Leg

The posterior thigh region is composed of the biceps femoris, the semi-tendinosis, and the semi-membranous. These muscles assist with extending the thigh and rotating the knee. The biceps femoris is more commonly known as the hamstrings, and is made up of the long head and the short head. The long head of the biceps femoris originates at the ischial tuberosity and the sacrotuberous ligament. It inserts on the lateral side of the fibula and the tibia. The short head originates at the lateral edge of the linea aspera, a rough ridge on the posterior portion of the fibula. Both of these help with the lateral rotation of the leg and hip. Other muscles that cause the leg to extend at the knee include the rectus femoris, vastus lateralis, vastus intermedius, and the vastus medialis.

MUSCLES THAT ACT ON THE FOOT

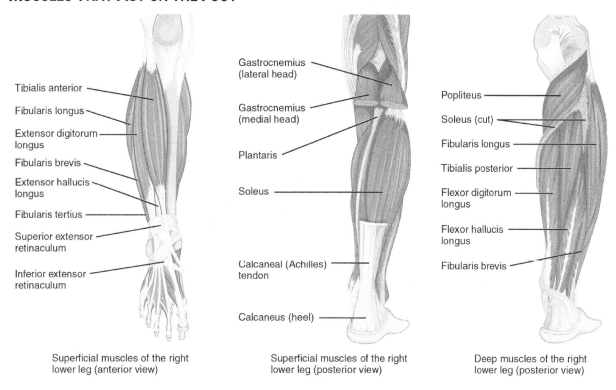

Superficial muscles of the right lower leg (anterior view)

Superficial muscles of the right lower leg (posterior view)

Deep muscles of the right lower leg (posterior view)

Kinesiology

The following is a list of muscles that act on the foot and cause moment as a result of inversion, extension, and flexion:

- **Popliteus** – responsible for medial rotation and flexion of the leg below the knee
- **Tibialis Anterior** – responsible for dorsiflexion and inversion
- **Peroneus Tertius** – responsible for dorsiflexion and eversion; not present in all people
- **Extensor Digitorum Longus** – responsible for dorsiflexion and eversion of the foot as well as extension of the toes
- **Extensor Hallucis Longus** – responsible for dorsiflexion and inversion of the foot, as well as extension of the big toe
- **Gastrocnemius** (Medial Head and Lateral Head) – responsible for flexing the knee during foot dorsiflexion and flexing the plantar during knee extension
- **Plantaris** – flexes the knee
- **Soleus** – responsible for plantar flexion
- **Flexor Digitorum Longus** – responsible for plantar flexion, inversion, and toe flexion
- **Flexor Hallucis Longus** – primarily responsible for plantar flexion, inversion, and toe flexion
- **Tibialis Posterior** – responsible for plantar flexion and inversion
- **Peroneus Longus** – responsible for eversion and plantar flexion
- **Peroneus Brevis** – responsible for eversion and plantar flexion

59

MUSCLES THAT ACT UPON THE ABDOMINAL REGION

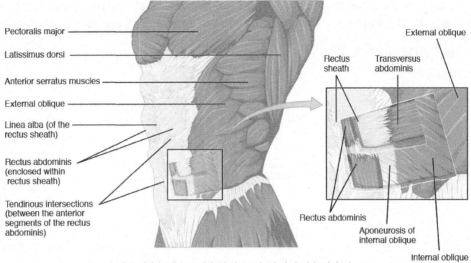

(a) Superficial and deep abdominal muscles (anterior lateral view)

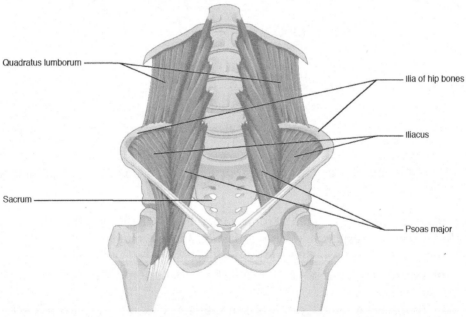

(b) Posterior abdominal muscles (anterior view)

Several muscle groups act upon the abdominal area. These include the rectus abdominis, which is responsible for flexing the trunk and tensing the abdominal walls. The external obliques run alongside the external surfaces of the lower eight ribs. These muscles extend from below the armpit down towards the waist. They allow for bilateral movement and the side to side rotation of the trunk. The internal obliques lie just underneath the external, and provide for the same movements as the external obliques. The transverse abdominis muscles lie underneath the rectus abdominis, and also help with flexion and compression of the abdominal wall. The rectus abdominis can be palpitated from the sternum down to the pubis. The external obliques can be felt on the lateral side of the abdomen. The internal obliques and the transverse abdominis are situated deep within the abdominal region; they cannot be palpitated.

MUSCLES THAT ASSIST IN THE RESPIRATORY PROCESS

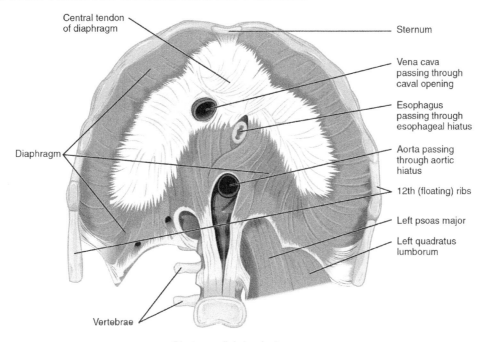

Diaphragm (inferior view)

The primary muscle used to assist with the respiratory process is the diaphragm. It is located between the upper lumbar vertebrae and within the region of the six lowest ribs and costal cartilage. The diaphragm has no insertion point. The main purpose of the diaphragm is to contract the muscles used for inspiration (the intake of air). The muscle cannot readily be palpitated, but can be seen during the respiratory process. Other respiratory muscles include the intercostals, which are made up of the external, internal, and innermost components. These muscles are located between each of the ribs, and serve to pull apart the ribs during inspiration, allowing for greater lung capacity. The serratus posterior superior, located near the collarbone, and the serratus posterior inferior, located at the base of the ribs, serve to expand the ribs outwards and downwards, which also leads to an increase in lung capacity.

Kinesiology

MUSCLE GROUPS THAT PROVIDE FOR LATERAL EXTENSION, FLEXION, STABILIZATION, AND ROTATION OF THE SPINE

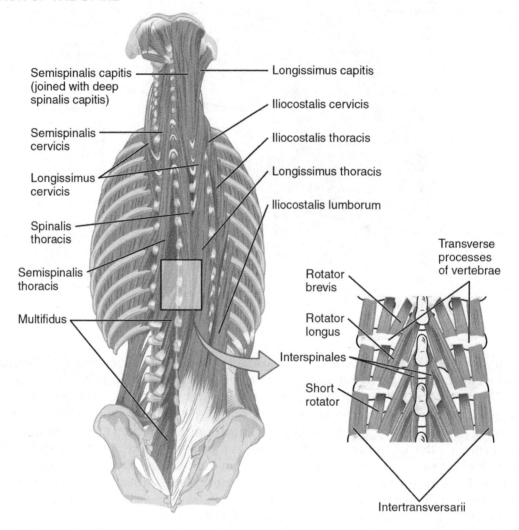

The following is a list of the muscles that run alongside the spinal column. All are difficult to palpitate through the skin.

- **Quadratus Lumborum** – responsible for lateral flexion of the spine
- **Intertransversarii** – located between the transverse processes of the vertebrae
- **Interspinales** – found in pairs located on either side of the contiguous vertebrae
- **Rotatores** – located only in the thoracic region; assists in flexion of the spine
- **Multifidus** – assists in the rotation of the spine
- **Semispinalis** – (includes capitis, cervicis, and thoracis); longitudinal muscles connected to the vertebrae
- **Spinalis** – (includes capitis, cervicis, and thoracis); bundled with a group of tendons and directly next to the spine
- **Longissimus** – (includes capitis, cervicis, and thoracis); help to extend the vertebral column, flex the spine laterally, and rotate the head and neck to either side

MUSCLES THAT AID IN MASTICATION

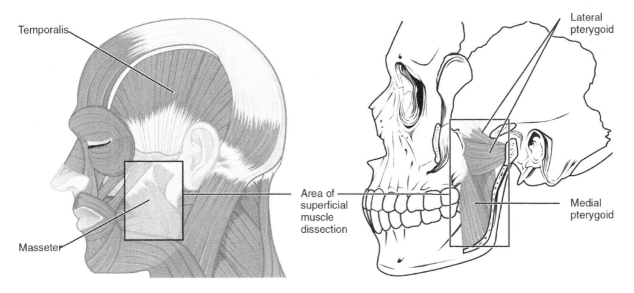

Chewing muscles (superficial)   Chewing muscles (deep)

Mastication is defined as the act of chewing, which is the process by which the teeth break food down into smaller particles that are easily swallowed. Many muscles aid this process. The masseter is responsible for closing the jaw, and can be found near the zygomatic arch and the mandible. The temporalis, which originates at the temporal bone, causes the jaw to close and retract. The buccinator, which originates at the maxilla and mandible, helps to keep the cheeks close to the teeth to allow the food to remain in place for chewing. The internal pterygoid helps to close the jaw and move the jaw from side to side. The external pterygoid causes the lower jaw to protrude forward, an action associated most often with an under bite.

MUSCLES THAT AID IN THE MOVEMENT OF THE EYE

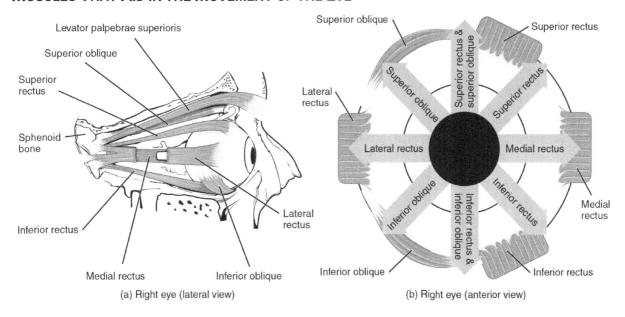

(a) Right eye (lateral view)   (b) Right eye (anterior view)

Kinesiology

The muscles of the eye provide for side-to-side and up-and-down movement. They allow a person to focus on objects without moving their head. None of these muscles can be palpitated. The eye muscles are as follows:

- **Levator Palpebrae Superioris** – Causes the eyelid to open
- **Superior Oblique** – Causes the eye to turn out and downwards
- **Superior Rectus** – Causes the eye to rotate upwards
- **Lateral Rectus** – Causes lateral movement
- **Inferior Rectus** – Moves the eye downwards
- **Medial Rectus** – Moves the eye medially
- **Inferior Oblique** – Moves the eye upwards and out

MUSCLES THAT AID IN THE FORMATION OF FACIAL EXPRESSIONS

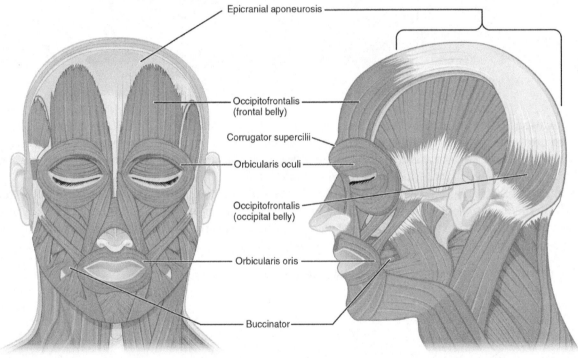

Facial muscles (anterior view)   Facial muscles (lateral view)

The muscles that are used to form the facial expressions associated with happiness, sadness, anger, etc. are aided by the following muscle groups:

- **Epicranius** – (also known as the occipitofrontalis); runs from the occipital bone to the frontal bone; helps to raise the eyebrow
- **Corrugator** – lowers the medial end of the eyebrow and wrinkles the brow
- **Procerus** – originates from the membrane that covers the bridge of the nose; assists the motion of the frontal bone
- **Orbicularis Oculi** – lowers the eyelids
- **Nasalis** – compresses the cartilage of the nose
- **Dilator Naris** – helps to manipulate the nostrils
- Quadratus Labii Superioris – raises the upper lip
- **Zygomaticus** – moves the mouth up and back
- **Orbicularis Oris** – puckers the lips

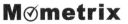

- **Risorius** – brings the edges of the mouth backwards; associated with a smile or grimace
- **Depressor Anguli Oris** – lowers the angle of the mouth
- Depressor Labii Inferioris – lowers the lower lip
- **Mentalis** – responsible for movement of the mouth back and down; associated with a frown
- **Platysma** – draws the lower lip down, wrinkling the neck and upper chest
- **Auricularis** – wiggles the ears

MUSCLES THAT AID IN THE MOVEMENT OF THE FOREHEAD

The muscle groups that assist the body perform movements such as frowning, drawing the eyebrows together, wrinkling the forehead, and drawing the nose upwards are listed below:

- **Epicranius** (consisting of the occipitalis and frontalis) – This muscle originates just above the occipital ridge and inserts at the epicranial aponeurosis. This muscle draws the epicranius towards the back, or posterior, of the head. It also raises the eyebrows, which causes the forehead to wrinkle. This muscle is sometimes known as the occipitofrontalis.
- **Corrugator** – This muscle is also known as the corrugator supercilii. It is triangular in shape and is responsible for wrinkling the forehead and also for the action of frowning.
- **Procerus** – The origin of this muscle is within the fascia over the cartilage in the nasal area. It inserts between the eyebrows and deep within the skin. This muscle is responsible for the action of wrinkling the nose.

MUSCLES THAT AID IN THE MOVEMENT OF THE EYES AND NOSTRILS

The muscles that are involved with this region of the face include:

- **Orbicularis Oculi** – Controls the opening and closing of the eye. This muscle originates at the nasal bone and circles the eyeball. The insertion point of this muscle is all around the eye; the muscle blends in with the surrounding areas.
- **Nasalis** – This muscle originates above the incisors at the maxilla bone. It then blends in with the procerus muscle. The purposes of this muscle are to compress the bridge of the nostrils, allow the external area of the nostrils to elevate, or flare, and also to depress the tip of the nose.
- **Dilator Naris** – This muscle allows the nostril opening to expand. It originates at the greater alar cartilage and inserts at the end point of the nose.

MUSCLES RESPONSIBLE FOR MOVING THE MOUTH

There are about eight muscle groups that are responsible for the various movements of the mouth. They include:

- **Quadratus Labii Superioris** – This lies next to the nose and extends to the zygomatic arch. It is responsible for raising or elevating the upper lip.
- **Zygomaticus** (major and minor) – This muscle extends from one side of the zygomatic arch to the corner of the mouth. The contraction of this muscle causes the mouth to draw back and upwards; this movement is associated with smiling.
- **Orbicularis Oris** – This muscle originates from various muscles around the mouth and inserts at the lips. It is a circular muscle that allows the mouth to remain closed, aids in chewing, helps with speech, and aids in the formation of facial expressions.
- **Risorius** – This muscle originates over the masseter. It inserts at the muscle surrounding the mouth and at the corners of the mouth. It is responsible for moving the mouth backwards at an angle.

65

- **Depressor Anguli Oris** – This muscle is responsible for drawing the mouth into a downward position, and is located at the outer edge of the chin.
- **Depressor Labii Inferioris** – This muscle helps to depress the lower lip.
- **Mentalis** – This muscle causes the chin to rise up and also enables a person to pout.
- **Platysma** – This muscle causes the mouth to move in a downward direction, enabling a person to form an expression of sadness. It also causes the skin of the neck to wrinkle.

PROPRIOCEPTION

Proprioception is the body's ability to gauge its own position in the external world. At all times, we are engaged in unconscious acts of proprioception that allow us to move around in harmony with our surroundings. Proprioception is often referred to as spatial orientation. Scientists believe that the human capacity for proprioception can be attributed to the endings of peripheral nerve fibers in the muscles and joints. The information that is obtained from these nerve endings is integrated with information from other sources, including the visual, auditory, tactile, and vestibular systems. The vestibular system senses the velocity of head movements and the relative pull of gravity on the body, and can therefore provide important information about the orientation of the body.

TREATING MUSCLE SPASMS

A muscle spasm is a dysfunction of the muscle in which involuntary contractions occur in a single muscle or a group of muscles. The intensity of these spasms can vary depending on the person's pain tolerance and how long the contractions continue. These spasms are classified as tonic when they remain in a contracted state for an extended time, and as clonic when the spasm relaxes between contractions. Another term for a muscle spasm is cramp. Typical kinds of spasms include hiccups, charley horses, twitches, and convulsions. Muscles can also spasm as a result of nearby injuries. When treating a spasm, massaging the area directly is not recommended until the acute spasm has subsided. It is thought that compressing the ends of the muscle or preventing the contraction of the antagonist muscles will help quiet the muscle spasm. Massaging the area after the acute phase has passed will help eliminate toxins from the muscle, introduce nutrients to the area, and restore circulation.

MUSCLE STRAINS

The term muscle strains can also refer to torn or pulled muscles. There are generally three degrees of strains that can occur to the muscle. A grade 1 strain is when the muscle fibers have been overextended, but there are very few tears in the fibers. There is pain, but there are no visual marks on the surface of the skin. There is also no loss of muscle function. When a grade 2 strain occurs, there are partial tears in less than 50% of the muscle fibers. There is pain, tenderness, inflammation, and loss of function to some degree. A grade 3 strain is when more than 50% of the muscle fibers are torn. There is considerable pain, and the bleeding may be seen under the skin. Swelling and immediate loss of muscle function occurs. Recovering from these types of injuries usually involves the use of the R.I.C.E. method (rest, ice, compression, and elevation) and massage once the acute stage has passed. It is important to maintain a good range of motion and flexibility once this stage is over to prevent muscle atrophy and reduce scarring.

HYPERTROPHY AND ATROPHY

It is possible for muscles to increase in size and get larger. As seen in bodybuilders, the size of the muscle increases through repeated strength training. This increase in the width of a muscle is known as hypertrophy. The muscular fibers themselves do not increase in number. Rather, the width of the muscle fibers increases. This increase causes the body part affected by the muscle to grow stronger. It will have more power while performing required actions or movements. Other changes that occur are an increase in the blood supply to the hypertrophic muscle and also an increase in ATP and mitochondria. Muscle atrophy refers to the degeneration and wasting away of muscles, which occurs as a result of disuse. Muscles that are not used break down and shrink, gradually losing their strength. The amount of blood supplied to the limb decreases, causing a change in the color of the limb. Atrophy commonly occurs in individuals with paralysis who have lost nerve connections to the muscles, which causes them to waste away.

TENDONITIS, TENOSYNOVITIS, AND LUPUS

Tendonitis is the condition in which the tendon that connects the muscle to the bone becomes inflamed. Tenosynovitis is the inflammation that occurs along the tendon sheath. Both of these conditions cause pain, stiffness, and swelling of the affected area. Treatment regimens include massage over the inflamed area, the application of ice to decrease swelling, and physical manipulation to increase range of motion and assist with prevention of scar tissue. Lupus is an autoimmune disease that can affect tissues and organs. This disease affects the connective tissue and can cause pain throughout many areas of the body. With this disease, blood vessels may become inflamed and arthritis can occur. Massage therapy on a person with lupus should be performed under the supervision of a physician to prevent pain to the patient.

FIBROMYALGIA AND MUSCULAR DYSTROPHY

Fibromyalgia is a disease that also affects connective tissue, producing pain, stiffness, and fatigue in the muscles, tendons, and ligaments. Factors such as temperature, humidity, and infections can cause an increase in the person's discomfort level and trigger additional symptoms. With the pain levels of each person varying, it is important to work with the client's personal physician to develop a massage plan. Muscular dystrophy is a disease that causes progressive degeneration of the muscles in the body. The muscular fibers are gradually replaced by fat and connective tissues, eventually leaving the muscle unable to function. If it does not induce pain, massage is beneficial in preventing the onset of muscle degeneration.

Joint Structure and Function

SYNOVIAL JOINT

The structures of a synovial joint are listed and described below:

- **Synovial cavity** - The synovial cavity is the space between the bones that are articulating at that joint.
- **Articular cartilage** – Articular cartilage covers the bones at a synovial joint. It is made up of hyaline cartilage or fibrocartilage. Articular cartilage is responsible for reducing friction between the bones and absorbing shock.
- **Articular capsule** – The articular capsule is a sleeve which surrounds the synovial joint. It encloses the joint and assists in articulation of the bones. It is composed of two layers, the fibrous capsule and the synovial membrane.
- **Fibrous capsule** – The fibrous capsule is the outer layer of the articular capsule. It attaches to the periosteum of the bones. The fibrous capsule is both flexible, which permits movement at the joint; and strong, which prevents dislocation.

Kinesiology

- **Synovial membrane** – The synovial membrane is the inner layer of the articular capsule. It contains flexible elastic fibers and secretes synovial fluid.
- **Synovial fluid** – Synovial fluid is secreted by the synovial membrane. Synovial fluid lubricates the joint to reduce friction and is also responsible for supplying nutrients and cleaning up debris in the joint due to wear and tear.

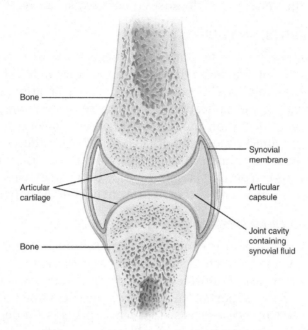

SYNARTHROTIC, AMPHIARTHROTIC, AND DIARTHROTIC JOINT CLASSIFICATIONS

Synarthrotic, amphiarthrotic, and diarthrotic are classifications of joints based on the amount of movement they permit. Joints classified as synarthrotic are considered immovable. An example of a synarthrotic joint would be the sutures in the skull. Amphiarthrotic joints are those which have limited motion. Examples of amphiarthrotic joints are the pubic symphysis and the sacroiliac joints. Diarthrotic joints are joints that move freely. They come in a variety of shapes and allow movement in various planes depending upon their structure. Diarthrotic joints have articular cartilage lining the ends of the bones that articulate at that joint and a joint capsule that consists of a synovial membrane that secretes synovial fluid.

TYPES OF SYNOVIAL JOINTS

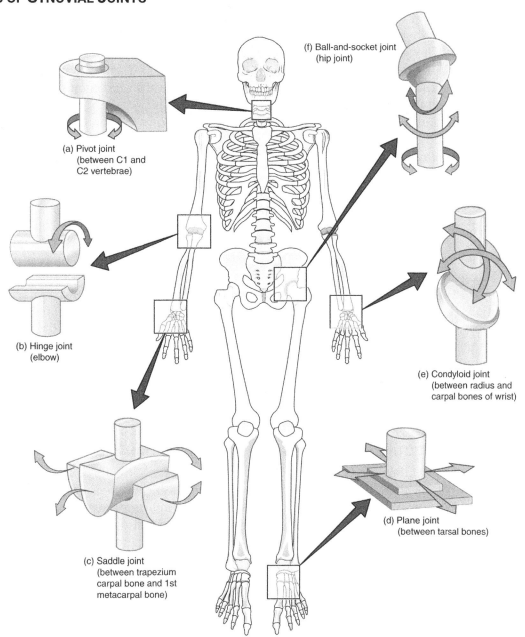

The types of synovial joints are listed and described below:

- **Hinge joints** have two articulating surfaces that fit together. One surface is convex and fits into the concave surface of the opposing bone. Together they allow the joint to move in an opening and closing action, much like the hinge of a door. The movements that occur at this joint would be flexion and extension. The knee joint is an example of a hinge joint.
- **Pivot joints** have a surface made up of bone and ligament which forms a ring into which the rounded or pointed surface of another bone will fit. This allows the joint to rotate around its axis. An example of a pivot joint would be the joint between axis and atlas which allows the head to rotate.

- **Condyloid joints** have two oval-shaped articulating surfaces, one convex and the other concave, which fit together and allow the joint to move in two planes. An example is the articulation at the wrist which is able to move up and down and side-to-side.
- **Saddle joints** have an articulating surface that is saddle shaped and allows the other articulating surface to sit on it like a rider would sit on a horse. A saddle joint allows for movement both side-to-side and up and down. An example of a saddle joint is the joint between the thumb and wrist metacarpals.
- **Ball-and-socket joints** have a cup-like depression that allows the ball-like articulating surface of another bone to fit inside. Ball-and-socket joints are considered multiaxial, which means they allow movement in three planes. Examples would be the shoulder and hip joints.

HYPERMOBILE AND HYPOMOBILE

A joint is described as hypermobile when it has an unusually large range of motion. This is sometimes referred to as being "double-jointed" or having loose joints. For most people, this will cause no problems and could even be beneficial to dancers and athletes. Hypermobility is often hereditary and commonly occurs in multiple joints. The joint will feel very loose and springy during range of motion testing. A joint is referred to as hypomobile when it has a smaller than normal range of motion. The biggest problem with a hypomobile joint is that it will cause other joints above and below it to compensate for the lack of movement. This can often lead to injury. Hypomobility is caused by ligaments that are too short and lack the necessary flexibility. The muscles may be tight as well. Attempting to overstretch a hypomobile joint will cause injury and pain and should be avoided.

Range of Motion

OBJECTIVE AND SUBJECTIVE FINDINGS DURING RANGE OF MOTION TESTING

When testing range of motion, the practitioner should be looking for both objective and subjective findings. Objective findings can be seen or felt by the practitioner and are measurable. Subjective findings are those that cannot be seen or felt, but the client may report or the practitioner may notice. Examples of objective findings would be decreased range of motion or abnormal end feels and the strength of the muscles being tested during a resistive test. Examples of subjective findings are the amount of pain felt during the movement, how the client reacts to the range of motion testing, and any other feedback the client may give. Both of these types of findings are important to note in order to properly assess and document any problems the client may be having with their range of motion. These findings can also be compared to future findings to assess whether the treatment protocol has been effective.

CONTRACTILE AND INERT TISSUE

Contractile and inert are two types of classifications for soft tissue. The primary difference between the two is their ability to activate and produce movement. Contractile tissues produce movement. Inert tissues do not have contractile properties. Muscle and tendon are contractile tissue. Nerves, bursa, fascia, and ligaments are all inert tissues. Even though inert tissues do not produce movement, they do move during muscle contraction. When a client is performing an active movement at a joint, both contractile and inert tissues are involved. When the practitioner is performing a passive range of motion test, the inert tissues are emphasized. This is due to the fact that the contractile tissue is not activated by muscular activity. Understanding the difference between these two types of tissues is important to the assessment process. If a client has pain during an active movement, it is possible that either or both contractile and inert tissues are

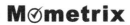

involved. If a client only feels pain during a passive range of motion test, then it is most likely that inert tissues are involved.

ASSESSING RANGE OF MOTION

Testing range of motion is one of the ways of assessing the condition of a client's tissue and can be used to determine a treatment plan and also to track progress and the success of treatment. By evaluating a joint's range of motion, a practitioner is able to identify which tissues are involved, the severity of the issue, and determine if other more appropriate therapies are advised before beginning massage. As treatment progresses with a client, a practitioner is able to do additional range of motion testing to evaluate the effectiveness of the treatments and ensure that the client is seeing improvement. If there is no improvement, the practitioner can adjust the treatment plan or refer the client out for further evaluation. Testing range of motion also gives the client a visual representation of how the treatments are helping them. If a practitioner is billing insurance for the services rendered, then range of motion testing is a valuable way to show objective results from the treatment.

The steps in testing active range of motion are as follows:

1. Determine the motions possible at the joint being evaluated.
2. Select the motion to be evaluated. It is best to perform single plane movements one at a time in order to best assess the condition of the joint. If any movements are painful, have the client perform those movements last to avoid irritation.
3. Determine which tissues are involved in the motion. It is important for the practitioner to understand which muscles are being used in order to have an accurate assessment.
4. Instruct the client on how to perform the movement. It helps to demonstrate to the client which movements you would like them to complete.
5. Have the client perform the movement. If the client has a complaint on one side, only have them complete the movement on the unaffected side first so as to evaluate the normal pain-free range of motion.
6. Take note of the quality movement. Look for pain or decreased range of motion.

Passive range of motion test is performed as follows:

1. Determine the motions possible at the joint being evaluated.
2. Select the motion to be evaluated. Be sure to test any movements that were painful during passive range of motion testing. Complete each single plane movement one at a time.
3. Determine which tissues are involved. During passive movement, the inert tissue is being activated. Be aware, however, that opposing muscles may be hypertonic and limit the range of motion.
4. Determine the normal end feel. It is important to have an understanding of what the typical end feel is like at the joint being tested.
5. Have the client relax as much as possible and allow the practitioner to perform the movement.
6. Perform the passive movement. Be sure to check the uninvolved side first to determine if there are symptoms on only one side of the body. Feel for any restrictions that may be preventing full range of motion.
7. Take notes of any pain or restrictions.

71

The steps taken in performing a resistive range of motion test are as follows:

1. Determine the motions possible at the joint being evaluated.
2. Select the motion to be evaluated. All movements at the joint should be tested. If any movements are painful during active movement, then they should be tested last to prevent irritation.
3. Determine which tissues are involved. Inert tissue will be involved in all movements, but the contractile tissue involved will vary based on the movement.
4. Find a position that effectively engages the desired muscle or muscles. It is best to test the muscle when it is in the middle of its range of motion as compared to being in a fully extended or flexed position, which is more taxing.
5. Have the client perform a contraction against resistance. This can be done by placing the client in the appropriate position, then instructing the client to maintain that position against force, not allowing any movement. If the client is unable to complete this task, then it would indicate a weakness in the muscle.
6. Make note of any findings. Weakness in a muscle should be documented as part of the assessment process.

Pathology, Contraindications, Areas of Caution, and Special Populations

Overview of Pathologies

ASTHMA, CHRONIC BRONCHITIS, PNEUMONIA, AND COLD

The pathologies, their common symptoms, and their relevance to massage therapy are discussed below:

- **Asthma** – tightening of the bronchial tubes; results in wheezing, coughing, and trouble breathing; massage can help to strengthen the muscles involved in breathing
- **Chronic bronchitis** – inflammation and infection of the bronchi; often occurs in conjunction with emphysema; massage can be helpful, so long as the patient is monitored closely
- **Pneumonia** – inflammation of the lungs; manifests as fever, chills, chest pain, cough, and difficulty breathing; massage is beneficial once the patient has passed out of the acute phase
- **Cold** – viral infection of the upper respiratory tract; symptoms can include fever, coughing, mucus overproduction, and headache; massage is helpful for managing symptoms and strengthening the immune system

ATHEROSCLEROSIS, THROMBUS, EMBOLISM, AND HYPERTENSION

The pathologies, their common symptoms, and their relevance to massage therapy are discussed below:

- **Atherosclerosis** – hardening of the arteries; individuals with this condition should not receive rigorous circulatory massage
- **Thrombus** – a blood clot that remains fixed in the blood stream; massage is contraindicated
- **Embolism** – a blood clot that is moving through the bloodstream; massage is contraindicated
- **Emphysema** – hardening of the alveoli in the lungs; symptoms include trouble breathing, cough, and chronic respiratory infection; massage is alright, so long as the patient can breathe effectively and the condition is not acute
- **Hypertension** – high blood pressure in the pulmonary arteries; massage is indicated, so long as the individual is not suffering from kidney or cardiovascular conditions

BENIGN PROSTATIC HYPERPLASIA, ENDOMETRIOSIS, PERITONITIS, AND PROSTATITIS

The pathologies, their common symptoms, and their relevance to massage therapy are discussed below:

- **Benign prostatic hyperplasia** – irregular growth of the prostate gland; may cause problems with urination; does not prevent massage
- **Endometriosis** – overgrowth of endometrial cells in the peritoneal cavity; may lead to heavy menstruation, abdominal pain, and problems with intercourse and/or evacuation; massage is indicated, except in the affected area

- **Peritonitis** – inflammation of the membrane along the inner wall of the abdomen and pelvis; caused by infection or disease; manifests in severe abdominal pain; massage is contraindicated, and the client should receive immediate medical attention
- **Prostatitis** – inflammation of the prostate gland; may result in chills, fever, testicular pain, pain in the lower back, and difficulty with urination; circulatory massage is contraindicated if the patient is in the acute phase

BOILS, BUNIONS, BURNS, AND BEDSORES

The pathologies, their common symptoms, and their relevance to massage therapy are discussed below:

- **Boils** – bacterial infections on the skin; manifests as red sores; often appear in clusters; should not be massaged, especially because they may be quite contagious
- **Bunions** – a growth of the bone at the base of the big toe; should not be massaged
- **Burns** – may be first-degree (slight inflammation), second-degree (damage to epidermis), or third-degree (including damage to the dermis); once the burn has passed out of the acute stage, it may be massaged so long as it does not hurt
- **Bedsores** – lesions caused by impaired circulation; should not be massaged directly, although massage is a good way to prevent bedsores

FUNGAL INFECTIONS, HERPES, HIVES, AND LICE

The pathologies, their common symptoms, and their relevance to massage therapy are discussed below:

- **Fungal infections** – manifest on the skin as red, itchy patches and blisters; may result in the weakening and infection of finger and toe nails; massage is contraindicated at the site of the infection
- **Herpes** – a virus that causes lesions and blisters; contraindicated in the acute stage and when the client has an infection or outbreak; equipment that comes into contact with the client should be washed
- **Hives** – a raised, scratchy patch of skin; usually caused by an allergic reaction; during the acute phase, massage is contraindicated everywhere; after the acute phase passes, massage is only contraindicated in the area of the hives
- **Lice** – parasitic insects; most often found on the scalp; symptoms include itching, irritation, and sores; massage is contraindicated, especially because lice are highly contagious

MOLES, PSORIASIS, ULCERS, AND TENDINITIS

The pathologies, their common symptoms, and their relevance to massage therapy are discussed below:

- **Moles** – pigmented spots on the skin; moles should not affect the delivery of massage services; however, moles that change in color or shape should be reported to the client's doctor
- **Psoriasis** – a red, scaly skin rash; most often located on the elbows, knees, and scalp; not contagious; contraindicated locally during the acute phase; indicated during the subacute phase
- **Ulcers** – any lesion that is eroding the membrane or surrounding skin; massage is contraindicated locally
- **Tendinitis** – inflammation of a tendon; usually caused by injury; massage is indicated, especially for reducing inflammation

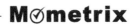

HIV/AIDS, Cystic Fibrosis, Cancer, and Multiple Sclerosis

The pathologies, their common symptoms, and their relevance to massage therapy are discussed below:

- **HIV/AIDS** – a disease that ravages the immune system; HIV becomes AIDS when it integrates into the DNA of the individual; massage is indicated so long as the client is in relatively good health
- **Cystic fibrosis** – disease which results in exceptionally thick production of mucus, sweat, bile, and other body products; symptoms may include problems with breathing, coughing, and lung infections; massage is indicated, unless the patient's symptoms preclude it
- **Cancer** – a growth of malignant cells; massage can be beneficial so long as it does not reduce the body's strength during a period of intense and debilitating treatments
- **Multiple sclerosis** – a permanent disease; manifests in symptoms like numbness, blindness, and paralysis; massage is indicated in the subacute phase

Depression, Headaches, Premenstrual Syndrome, and Fever

The pathologies, their common symptoms, and their relevance to massage therapy are discussed below:

- **Depression** – any diminution in quality of life, outlook, or happiness; massage can be extremely beneficial in mitigating the effects of depression
- **Headaches** – massage is indicated unless the headache is due to infection or damage to the central nervous system
- **Premenstrual syndrome** – a set of physical and psychological changes that occur directly before menstruation; symptoms can include breast tenderness, bloating, moodiness, and anger; bodywork can be especially beneficial while a woman is experiencing PMS
- **Fever** – slight increase in body temperature; massage is contraindicated; if a fever is greater than 102 degrees, the client should receive immediate physical attention

Varicose Veins, Warts, Cysts, and Lyme Disease

The pathologies, their common symptoms, and their relevance to massage therapy are discussed below:

- **Varicose veins** – enlarged and twisted veins; may result in cramps and trouble with movement; massage is contraindicated locally
- **Warts** – small growths on the outer layer of skin; contracted by contact with another wart; massage is contraindicated locally
- **Cysts** – pockets of connective tissue surrounding a foreign body; should not be massaged directly
- **Lyme disease** – an inflammatory disease caused by a bacterium transmitted by deer ticks; can result in a rash, symptoms of influenza, and pain in the joints; massage can improve joint function during subacute phases

Pathology, Contraindications, Areas of Caution, and Special Populations

75

CEREBRAL PALSY, MENINGITIS, AND MUSCULAR DYSTROPHY

The pathologies, their common symptoms, and their relevance to massage therapy are discussed below:

- **Cerebral palsy** – a family of injuries to the central nervous system; symptoms may include poor coordination, involuntary movements, and muscular disfiguration; massage can be very beneficial for individuals with cerebral palsy
- **Meningitis** – an inflammation of the membranes that surround the brain and spinal cord; can be caused by bacteria, protozoa, or viruses; massage is strictly contraindicated during the acute phase; once this passes massage can be beneficial
- **Muscular dystrophy** – a genetic disease in which the skeletal muscles gradually degenerate; may result in weakness, disability, and an inability to walk; massage can be quite effective at loosening muscles and improving circulation

BURSITIS, CARPAL TUNNEL SYNDROME, ENCEPHALITIS, AND PARKINSON'S DISEASE

The pathologies, their common symptoms, and their relevance to massage therapy are discussed below:

- **Bursitis** – inflammation in the areas where tendons, ligaments, and bones come into contact; when acute, massage is contraindicated; otherwise, there is no restriction on massage
- **Carpal tunnel syndrome** – irritation of the nerves in the hands; often caused by repetitive tasks; massage may be beneficial, especially around the wrist area
- **Encephalitis** – swelling of the brain; caused by infection; symptoms include fever, headache, and disorientation; massage only contraindicated if the condition is acute
- **Parkinson's disease** – degenerative neurological disease; manifests in expressionless face, involuntary movements, tremor, and muscle weakness; massage is indicated, so long as the movements of the client are respected

HEART ATTACK, HEART FAILURE, STROKE, AND GOUT

The pathologies, their common symptoms, and their relevance to massage therapy are discussed below:

- **Heart attack** – flow of blood through the heart is suddenly impeded; circulatory massage contraindicated during the recovery period
- **Heart failure** – heart is unable to supply enough blood to nourish the body; symptoms include lung fluid buildup, irregular pulse, and coughing; energetic massage is appropriate, but circulatory massage is strictly contraindicated
- **Stroke** – rapid death of brain cells; caused by a blockage of blood flow to the brain, which in turn results in an oxygen deficit; symptoms include loss of speech, weakness, and paralysis; all but the most vigorous circulatory massage is indicated for this group
- **Gout** – inflammation of the ankle and foot joints; feet and ankles will become swollen and painful; massage contraindicated

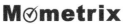

EDEMA, GALLSTONES, SCARIFICATION, AND PANCREATITIS

The pathologies, their common symptoms, and their relevance to massage therapy are discussed below:

- **Edema** – buildup of fluid between the organs; manifests in bloated areas on the body; in a severe, "pitting" edema, the body will not return to its natural form when pressure is applied; massage is contraindicated
- **Gallstones** – crystals made of hardened bile or cholesterol; massage indicated unless the client is in severe pain
- **Scarification** – buildup of scar tissue, as for instance over a wound; massage is contraindicated during the acute period
- **Pancreatitis** – inflammation of the pancreas; often caused by alcoholism or gallstones; symptoms include abdominal pain, nausea, vomiting, and fever; massage is appropriate once the condition has been thoroughly treated by a doctor

HERNIA, IRRITABLE BOWEL SYNDROME, TUBERCULOSIS, AND HEPATITIS

The pathologies, their common symptoms, and their relevance to massage therapy are discussed below:

- **Hernia** – small tear in the abdominal lining or inguinal ring; small intestine may poke through this hole; massage is contraindicated until the hernia has been treated
- **Irritable bowel syndrome** – an intestinal disorder in which the bowels and their nerves become over or under active; can manifest in abdominal pain, bloating, diarrhea, and constipation; massage is indicated; client should be monitored
- **Tuberculosis** – contagious infection; can only be identified by a chest x-ray
- **Hepatitis** – viral infection of the liver; massage is contraindicated when the disease is acute

DIABETES, HEMOPHILIA, HYPOGLYCEMIA, AND LUPUS

The pathologies, their common symptoms, and their relevance to massage therapy are discussed below:

- **Diabetes** – disorders of the metabolism; manifests in problems with appetite, urination, and blood sugar balance; massage is indicated unless the patient has specific circulation problems
- **Hemophilia** – condition in which the blood fails to clot normally; vigorous massage is contraindicated, though gentle techniques may be beneficial
- **Hypoglycemia** – low blood sugar; can manifest in anxiety, palpitations, sweating, and nausea; this condition is episodic, so if an individual is experiencing a bout of hypoglycemia, he or she should receive treatment before a massage
- **Lupus** – a disease in which chronic inflammation leads to degeneration of the immune system; can manifest in diseases of the skin, heart, lungs, kidneys, joints, and nervous system; massage is indicated so long as the client is not experiencing an acute episode

Pathology, Contraindications, Areas of Caution, and Special Populations

HERNIATED DISC, FRACTURES, OSTEOARTHRITIS, AND OSTEOARTHRITIS

The pathologies, their common symptoms, and their relevance to massage therapy are discussed below:

- **Herniated disc** – the matter between the vertebral discs is forced out, which puts pressure on the spinal cord and nerves; massage is indicated, so long as the condition is not acute
- **Fractures** – cracked or broken bones; massage contraindicated in the area of the fracture, though it can be beneficial elsewhere
- **Osteoarthritis** – gradual inflammation, disintegration, and loss of the joint cartilage; most often affects the feet, hands, spine, hips, and knees; during an acute inflammation, massage is strictly contraindicated
- **Osteoporosis** – reduction in bone mass; leads to a greater frequency of fracture; massage is indicated so long as the client is not in any great pain

URINARY TRACT INFECTION, HYPERTHYROIDISM, HYPOTHYROIDISM, AND RENAL FAILURE

The pathologies, their common symptoms, and their relevance to massage therapy are discussed below:

- **Urinary tract infection** – infection of the kidney, ureter, bladder, or urethra; symptoms may include painful urination and abdominal pain; circulatory massage is contraindicated during the acute phase; massage in the lower abdomen is contraindicated during the subacute phase
- **Hyperthyroidism** – excessive thyroid hormone production; can result in high heart rate, weight loss, and depression; massage can be beneficial, as it can reduce stress
- **Hypothyroidism** – deficiency of thyroid hormone; can result in fatigue, constipation, and weight gain; massage is indicated as it does not aggravate any accompanying atherosclerosis
- **Renal failure** – failure of the kidneys; may result in jaundice, edema, and even death; massage is systemically contraindicated during the acute and chronic phases

INFLUENZA, MONONUCLEOSIS, MYASTHENIA GRAVIS, AND SPINA BIFIDA

The pathologies, their common symptoms, and their relevance to massage therapy are discussed below:

- **Influenza** – virus of the respiratory tract; can result in fever, loss of appetite, and weakness; massage is only appropriate if the influenza has passed out of the acute phase
- **Mononucleosis** – a chronic infection; can last for one or two months; symptoms include fever, fatigue, sore throat, and swollen lymph nodes; massage is contraindicated during the acute phase
- **Myasthenia gravis** – an autoimmune neuromuscular disorder; manifests in extreme muscular fatigue; massage is indicated, though it will not improve the condition in any significant way
- **Spina bifida** – a birth defect in which part of the spine remains exposed; may result in incontinence, limited mobility, and learning difficulties; massage is indicated as part of a comprehensive physical therapy program

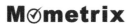

MENOPAUSE, RECOVERY FROM SURGERY, HEMATOMA, AND TREMORS

The pathologies, their common symptoms, and their relevance to massage therapy are discussed below:

- **Menopause** – the end of a woman's menstrual periods; usually diagnosed when a woman has not menstruated for one year; some related symptoms include mood swings, hot flashes, and fatigue; massage is extremely useful during menopause
- **Recovery from surgery** – the client should receive permission from his or her physician before receiving massage treatment
- **Hematoma** – deep intramuscular bruising; may or may not be visible externally; massage is contraindicated for acute hematoma; sub-acute hematoma may benefit from gentle circulatory massage
- **Tremor** – unnatural, repetitive shaking of the body; may be caused by illness, medication, or fear; massage is indicated

PLANTAR FASCIITIS, SHIN SPLINTS, AND MUSCLE SPASMS

The pathologies, their common symptoms, and their relevance to massage therapy are discussed below:

- **Plantar fasciitis** – inflammation of the tissue that stretches from the heel to the ball of the foot; symptoms include pain and difficulty walking; massage is indicated, as it can delay the formation of scar tissue and improve circulation in the calves
- **Shin splints** – inflammation of the tibia; results from overuse; manifests in pain; massage is indicated so long as the client does not have a stress fracture
- **Muscle spasms** – short, involuntary muscle contractions; caused by stress, medication, and overuse; massage around the muscle connector sites can improve the condition and reduce painful symptoms

DIAGNOSING AND TREATING A HERNIATED DISK

A herniated disk is an invertebral disk that has protruded out and into the spinal cavity, causing pain and increased pressure on the spinal cord. This disk can also cause pain and radiating pressure on the nerve endings leading down the legs. Most often occurring in the lumbar region, the typical herniated disk occurs gradually over time. When seeing a physician for this condition, diagnostic tests may be ordered to determine the degree of severity. These tests can include x-ray, myelogram, CT scan, and MRI to determine the exact cause of the pain; the symptoms can mimic other illnesses or diseases. Initial treatment of a herniated disk includes hot or cold therapy, massage, exercise, stretching, rest, pain medication, and, in severe or prolonged cases, surgery.

STRAIN AND SPRAIN

Strains and sprains are two of the most common muscular injuries. They may be severe and painful, or so minor as to be almost unnoticeable. A strain is an injury that occurs when a muscle has been stretched beyond its capabilities. It can also be referred to as a pulled muscle. Microscopic tears within the muscle cause pain, stiffness, swelling, and sometimes bruising. A sprain is an injury that occurs when a ligament is overstretched suddenly, causing pain, immediate swelling, and bruising. Severe sprains involve a popping, either felt or heard, and loss of function of that body part.

CLASSIFICATIONS OF SPRAINS

There are three main classifications of sprains. The first is identified as a class I sprain. This is when the ligament has been stretched, but there is little to no loss of limb function. The second is a class II sprain. The ligament is torn, and there is some loss of limb function. Some internal bleeding may

Pathology, Contraindications, Areas of Caution, and Special Populations

occur, or there may not be any bruising or discoloration. The third type, a class III sprain, involves a complete tear of the ligament, along with internal bleeding and extensive loss of function of the affected limb. All three types of sprains heal best when the R.I.C.E. method (rest, ice, compression, and elevation) is used. Massage is recommended only during the latent stages of healing, and will help prevent the formation of scars and increase range of motion and flexibility.

INFECTIONS

An infection within the body is an indication of the presence of microorganisms (such as bacteria, fungi, parasites, and viruses) that are capable of causing harm to the body. These microorganisms generally enter the body through cuts in the skin, through nasal passages, or by coming into contact with the bodily fluids of other individuals. The damage infections cause can range from simple, localized illnesses to diseases that ravage the entire body. Local infections are those that affect one small area of the body. If the infection has spread to other areas or all over the body, it is termed a systemic infection.

INFLAMMATION

It is important that massage techniques are not performed on localized areas that are infected or, in cases of systemic infection, on any part of the body. Inflammation can result from an infection, and causes five major changes to the body: redness, heat, swelling, pain, and loss of all or some function of the affected body part. Inflammation is an indicator of tissue damage. It is the result of an inflow of blood to the area and an increase in the production of white blood cells to aid in the healing process. It is important that these areas are not massaged while inflammation is present or while the patient has a fever.

CONTRAINDICATIONS TO MASSAGE

When performing a massage on a new client, it is important that the therapist obtain as thorough a medical history as possible. A contraindication is any procedure or treatment plan that, for the sake of the client's benefit and well-being, is not advisable. There are three types of contraindications that can exist: absolute, regional, or conditional. An absolute contraindication indicates that a massage should not be performed under any circumstances. Examples of this would include shock, pneumonia, and pregnancy-related toxemia. A regional contraindication exists when a client cannot have massage performed on a specific region of the body due to injuries, such as open wounds, contagious conditions that could cause harm to the therapist, or other conditions like arthritis. In the latter case, massage would result in additional pain to the client if the affected areas were massaged. The final type of contraindication is conditional. This means that the massage therapist must make accommodations in the therapeutic plan to help the client obtain the most benefit from the massage, while avoiding the areas that could cause discomfort.

HYPERTROPHY

Hypertrophy is an enlargement in a tissue or organ. Hypertrophy in muscle tissue is usually due to muscular resistance training. A muscle will grow in size due to repeated forceful activities. The hypertrophy is created by an increase in the size of the muscle fibers, not by an increase in the number of muscle fibers. The increase in size will strengthen the power of the muscle and increase blood supply, mitochondria, and ATP. Massage itself will not cause an enlargement in muscle tissue, but it can prevent atrophy, which is the loss of muscle tissue due to inactivity. Massage has been shown to help those who are bedridden, or who have suffered neurological injuries such as stroke, from losing muscle. Massage assists in these cases by providing an increased blood flow and nutrients to the muscle, which can prevent muscle tissue from atrophying. Massage can also assist an athlete who is trying to achieve hypertrophy in the muscles by removing metabolic waste and assisting with recovery, pain relief, and increasing range of motion.

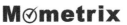

EDEMA

Edema is a condition in which there is excess fluid in the interstitial spaces, which are the spaces between organs or tissues. It is characterized by swelling and can often be felt by touch. Edema occurs due to an imbalance in the pressure of fluids within the capillaries. This can be caused by fluid retention from kidney malfunction, obstructions to the lymph vessels or veins, or changes in the capillary pressure. It is often associated with liver and kidney issues, a weakened heart, or injury or infection in the local area. Massage is usually a contraindication when there is kidney, liver, or heart involvement due to the overload of these systems when fluids are pushed through the body. Some massage can be used to treat edema in local tissues if there is no infection present. Lymph drainage massage is the recommended technique to use when edema is present and massage is indicated.

ISCHEMIA

Ischemia can happen to any tissue in the body. It is the state where blood flow has been inhibited to the tissue. It can cause serious damage, such as in a stroke when blood flow is cut off to brain tissue. In muscle tissue, ischemia is usually related to an injury. It can be as simple as a bruise or a mild muscle strain. When a muscle is injured, the reflex reaction is for the surrounding muscle tissue to contract in order to protect and support the injured tissue. This will constrict the blood vessels and capillaries in the area, preventing blood flow. Over time, due to metabolic processes, lactic acid and toxins will begin to build up in the area and collect in the tissue. This will cause ischemic pain in the muscle. Often this pain is more intense than the original injury. This can turn into a cycle of pain, followed by spasm, contraction of the muscle, followed by more pain. This is often why clients will seek massage for what was a minor injury that has become a more long-standing problem.

Contraindications

RASH ON THE THIGH

Rashes can be caused by a variety of reasons. The first step the practitioner should take is to ask the client if they are aware of the rash and what the cause is. The client may not be aware of the rash or may be under treatment. The practitioner should then let the client know that the thigh area will not be included in the massage due to the rash. If the client is aware of the rash and is under treatment, then when the rash is clear, the thigh area will again be included in the massage. If the client is not aware of the rash or is not undergoing treatment for it, the practitioner should recommend that the client seek medical advice. Once the rash is cleared, it would be acceptable to return to full massage in the area unless otherwise advised by the client's physician.

ATHLETE'S FOOT

Athlete's foot is a fungal infection that can be easily spread. It is often spread by walking barefoot in warm, moist areas such as pools or locker room shower areas. It most often presents as a moist, white, cracked area between the toes, but can also appear as red, scaly patches on the feet. Fungal infections can be difficult to treat. Athlete's foot would be considered a local contraindication and the feet should be avoided during massage. It can be spread through contact, so the massage practitioner should be careful not to allow any lubricant to come in contact with the affected area and should wash and sanitize the hands thoroughly after massaging a client with athlete's foot. A massage practitioner who is immunocompromised or pregnant may want to consider whether massaging a client with athlete's foot is appropriate due to the higher likelihood of it being spread in those conditions. Extra caution would be warranted in those situations.

Pathology, Contraindications, Areas of Caution, and Special Populations

BOILS

Boils are staphylococcus infections in sebaceous glands that have become clogged by dirt and debris. Boils are very similar to acne and the treatment protocol is similar, but more caution should be used. The staphylococcus bacterium that causes boils is extremely contagious and is often resistant to drug intervention. If a client presents with a boil and does not show any other signs of systemic infection, then massage would be indicated, however the area around the boil should be strictly avoided. If the client shows any signs of systemic infection, which includes fever, swelling of lymph nodes, or pain at sites other than the boil, then massage is not indicated. After massaging a client with a boil, there is a chance of contamination of the sheets. The practitioner must take extra care to isolate the sheets that are used during that massage and wash them separately in a 10 percent bleach solution. Also, any lubricants used during the massage that may have come in contact with the boil should be disposed of and hands must be sanitized immediately after the massage session.

CONTACT DERMATITIS

Dermatitis is a generic term for skin inflammation. Contact dermatitis is a skin irritation caused by an external stimulus. These types of irritations are usually caused by an immune system that is hypersensitive. People will commonly have reactions to laundry detergents, soaps, or other chemicals in their environment. Poison ivy and poison oak are also forms of contact dermatitis. Whether to massage or not is dependent on the cause of the irritation and the severity of the reaction. If the skin is very inflamed or blistered, then massage would be at least locally contraindicated, as long as there are no other symptoms. In the case of poison ivy or poison oak, or any type of rash that could spread, massage would be contraindicated due to the risks of spreading the rash. Dermatitis that is contained to a small area, such as irritation from a piece of jewelry, would be acceptable to massage as long as the immediate area of the dermatitis is avoided.

OSTEOPOROSIS

Osteoporosis is a condition which leads to the deterioration of bone, most commonly seen in the elderly. When this condition becomes advanced, the bones may become brittle and easily broken. Someone with osteoporosis may present with stooped shoulders or appear frail. It is often caused in women by decreasing estrogen levels. If a client with osteoporosis would like to receive massage, it is best that the practitioner consults with the client's physician regarding the safety of massage and whether it is indicated in this individual situation. If the physician approves of massage, then the practitioner will need to adjust the pressure level to avoid damage to the bones. A client with osteoporosis will often be frail and getting on to or off of the massage table may be a problem. The practitioner may need to assist the client with this or ask a family member or someone accompanying them to assist. Excessive joint movements should also be avoided due to the frailty of the bone structure.

CANCER

A practitioner treating a client with cancer should be working with the client's treatment team and have a full understanding of the type of cancer and current treatments. A new client should have a referral from a physician stating what types of massage are advised and any treatment considerations or contraindications. If the client has come to the appointment without a referral from the treating physician, the practitioner should defer the massage until that referral is received. If the client does have a referral, then the practitioner should do a thorough intake to learn the current status of the client, including type of cancer, what treatments are currently being used, as well as how the client is feeling that day. The practitioner should then follow the recommendations of the physician and create a treatment plan that both practitioner and client are comfortable with.

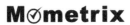

All guidelines for treating a client with cancer should be followed and the practitioner should contact the physician with any questions or concerns.

GUIDELINES

Before beginning a massage on someone with cancer, a complete medical history should be taken and a recommendation for massage should be received from the physician. A treatment plan should be developed and the client should give full consent. During the massage, lighter pressure should be used and sessions should be shorter to prevent fatigue. Deep tissue massage would be contraindicated. Massage to the tumor area or lymph nodes would also be contraindicated. If there are probable secondary metastatic sites, those should be avoided. No massage should be given when there is infection or fever. Consult with the client on their current state of health and adjust the massage accordingly. Depending on the treatment schedule, the client may have days that are better or worse than others. Getting feedback is important. Be aware of low blood counts that could be present and know the location of any ports. If the client is receiving radiation, there may be burns or sensitive areas that need to be avoided. Due to any recent surgery, there may be an increased risk of blood clots. Be sure to consult the client's physician with any questions or concerns.

FEVER

Normal body temperature is 98.6 degrees Fahrenheit or 37 degrees Celsius. General guidelines say that a temperature above 99.4 degrees Fahrenheit would be a contraindication for massage. The reason that massage is contraindicated in fever is due to the fact that fever is the body's way of isolating and eliminating an invading pathogen. When a microorganism such as bacteria invades the body, a reaction is started that will allow the body to fight off the invader. Part of that reaction is an increased core temperature. If a client has a fever, it is a red flag that the body is being invaded by a pathogen and the natural body systems should be allowed to run their course. The massage practitioner should not interfere with the body's natural regulatory system or alter the blood flow, as with massage. The fever will reach its crisis point and then begin to return to normal. The fever will also increase the heart rate, which will increase the distribution of white blood cells throughout the body. Massage during a fever may allow the pathogen to spread to the practitioner who could then spread this to other clients.

VARICOSE VEINS

Varicose veins are distended superficial veins. They often look twisted or rope-like and most often occur in the legs. They are caused by damage to the internal valves that control the flow of blood back to the heart. The blood should only flow in one direction but when the valves become damaged, the blood flows back into the veins and pools, causing distention. The most common cause of varicose veins is being on the feet for long periods of time. Women are more prone to varicose veins than men. Varicose veins will appear bluish in color and lumpy. Sometimes they are only visible while standing. There may also be edema due to the slowing of circulation. Most of the time, there is little or no pain involved, but there can be complications. Some people with varicose

Pathology, Contraindications, Areas of Caution, and Special Populations

veins will also develop eczema in the area. Severe cases may require surgery to prevent further health complications.

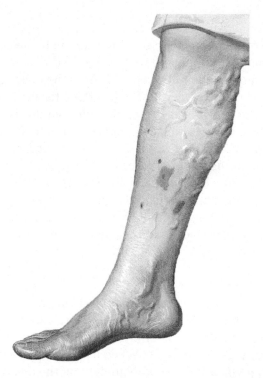

PERIPHERAL NEUROPATHY

Peripheral neuropathy is damage to the peripheral nerves. It is generally caused by some other disease or illness, usually diabetes or alcoholism. There can be sensory or motor damage or both. Burning or tingling pain and loss of movement are common symptoms. Peripheral neuropathy would be at least a local contraindication for massage. If a client is having symptoms of peripheral neuropathy but does not have a diagnosis, then a referral to a physician is recommended and massage would be contraindicated until the cause of the neuropathy has been identified. Peripheral neuropathy can cause the client to be either extremely sensitive to touch, which would make the massage uncomfortable; or there could be reduced sensation, which would make it difficult for the client to offer feedback on pressure. With any type of symptoms of peripheral neuropathy, the massage would be locally contraindicated and, depending on the reason for the neuropathy massage, may also be an absolute contraindication. That is why it is important to understand the client's entire health history before beginning massage.

MULTIPLE SCLEROSIS

Multiple sclerosis is a progressive disease that is characterized by inflammation and then gradual degeneration of the myelin sheaths in the brain and spinal cord. There are a wide variety of symptoms that can be present and the disease can go into remission then relapse. There are acute and subacute stages of the disease. Massage is indicated during the subacute stage. It is very important for the practitioner to use caution and not overstimulate a client with multiple sclerosis. This can cause painful, uncontrolled muscle spasms. The symptoms of multiple sclerosis are exacerbated by heat, so hydrotherapy or other therapies requiring heat would be contraindicated. If a client has sensation, then general massage can be applied in the area to prevent spasticity and maintain the health of the tissue. If the client does not have sensation, then very light effleurage or energy work would be advised to help keep some neurons firing. The practitioner should also check

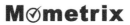

with a client about mobility issues and inquire if assistance will be needed getting on to and off of the massage table.

PRENATAL MASSAGE

A pregnant woman should receive permission from her doctor before receiving massage. Massage would be contraindicated if the woman is experiencing morning sickness, nausea, and diarrhea or has any type of vaginal discharge or bleeding. If there is high blood pressure, excessive swelling in the arms or legs, or if a decrease in fetal movement has been noticed, then massage would be contraindicated and an immediate referral to a physician would be recommended. If a woman is experiencing high blood pressure and edema, then massage would be definitely contraindicated and medical care should be sought immediately. Varicose veins are a common problem during pregnancy. Light effleurage can be done on the area around the varicose veins, but not directly over them. A pregnant woman is at greater risk of blood clots, so deep massage on the legs should be avoided during pregnancy. If there are any signs of blood clot such as redness, swelling, and tenderness in the legs, it is recommended that medical attention be sought immediately. If there are any health concerns present during pregnancy, a doctor's permission should be obtained before performing any type of massage.

FRAIL ELDERLY CLIENTS

A frail elderly client can benefit from massage but care must be taken during treatment. The elderly have delicate tissues and the skin would be susceptible to bruising and damage. The client may need assistance with dressing and may require help to get on and off the massage table. Ask the client if any assistance is needed. It is best not to massage frail elderly clients in the prone position. A side-lying position is usually best or the massage may have to be done in a seated position in a chair. If doing a home call, the client may be most comfortable being massaged in bed. Range of motion and joint movements should be done with extreme caution, especially if there is osteoporosis present. Sessions with frail elderly clients may need to be shorter than normal due to fatigue and all strokes should be gentler with light pressure and less gliding. A frail elderly client may also be under the care of a physician and on multiple medications. Ask if assistance is needed completing forms and look for contraindications that may be present. With frail elderly clients, it is better to do too little than too much.

PARALYSIS

People who have suffered paralysis, either through illness or injury, require certain special considerations. The massage practice must be wheelchair accessible to provide access to clients who may be using a mobility aid such as a wheelchair, scooter, or crutches. The first thing that must be decided is whether to have the client transfer onto the massage table or if the work is being done in a wheelchair or other location. If the client needs assistance on to the massage table, the practitioner must decide if it will be within their own physical and safety capabilities. If the table can be lowered to wheelchair height, this may be helpful. Be sure to use bolsters to make the client as comfortable as possible. If the client will remain in the wheelchair during massage, make sure to lock the wheels so there is no rolling. When massaging the part of the body that is paralyzed, the most important consideration is the loss of sensation. The client will not be able to give feedback on pressure, so deep techniques and joint movements should be avoided. The part of the body that is not paralyzed may receive general massage as normal.

HYDROTHERAPY TOOLS THAT RAISE THE CORE BODY TEMPERATURE

Contraindications for using hydrotherapy tools that raise the core body temperature:

- High or low blood pressure
- Heart or circulatory problems
- Pregnancy
- Seizures
- Multiple sclerosis
- Infections and fever
- Vascular problems associated with phlebitis, varicose veins, diabetes
- Skin rashes
- Contagious illnesses
- Some cancers and cancer treatments

HYDROTHERAPY TOOLS THAT LOWER THE CORE BODY TEMPERATURE

Conditions where hydrotherapy tools that lower core body temperature should not be used:

- People with Raynaud's phenomenon, a disorder where the blood vessels in the extremities constrict in cold; or any other circulatory insufficiency
- Cold sensitivity
- Multiple sclerosis
- Asthma
- Infection
- Depression
- Pregnancy
- Cardiac impairment

APPLICATION OF HEAT TO THE HEAD OR NECK FOR MIGRAINE HEADACHES

Migraine is a type of vascular headache that can cause varying symptoms, including severe throbbing pain, sensitivity to light and sound, nausea, and vomiting. The cause of migraine is not known exactly, but there are many triggers that can cause a migraine to begin. It is believed that migraine is caused when vessels on the surface of the brain dilate and create pressure on the nerves, causing intense pain. The application of heat is also a vasodilator and increases blood flow to the area where the heat is applied. Applying heat to the head and neck for migraine headache would only serve to increase the blood flow to the brain, possibly prolonging or increasing the symptoms. If the headache is being caused by muscle tension, then the application of heat could help in relaxing the muscles. In general, with a migraine headache, the best treatment would be the application of cold, while applications of heat would be contraindicated.

JOINT MOVEMENTS

Joint movements would be contraindicated in the following populations:

- Pregnant women due to the relaxation of ligaments from pregnancy hormones to prepare for birth
- Anyone with osteoporosis due to the risk of injury
- Frail elderly clients due to the risk of injury—may be done with extreme care
- Paralysis due to loss of sensation and risk of injury
- In cancer patients and the critically ill, joint movements should be avoided due to fatigue

Areas of Caution

ENDANGERMENT SITES ON THE BODY

The following are endangerment sites on the body:

- **Inferior to the ear** – The facial nerve, external carotid artery, and styloid process are all located in the notch posterior to the mandible and can be compressed and damaged.
- **Anterior triangle of the neck** – This area is bordered by the mandible, sternocleidomastoid muscle, and the trachea. The carotid artery, internal jugular vein, vagus nerve, and lymph nodes are all located in this triangle and should be avoided.
- **Posterior triangle of the neck** – This area is bordered by the sternocleidomastoid muscle, the trapezius muscle, and the clavicle and contains the brachial plexus, subclavian artery, brachiocephalic vein, external jugular vein, and lymph nodes.
- **Axilla** – The axilla is the armpit area and contains the axillary, ulnar, musculocutaneous, and median nerves; the axillary artery; and lymph nodes.
- **Medial brachium** – This area is located on the upper inner arm between the biceps and triceps. The medial brachium contains the ulnar, musculocutaneous, and median nerves; the brachial artery; basilica vein; and lymph nodes.
- **Cubital area of the elbow** – The cubital area is at the anterior bend of the elbow. This area contains the median nerve, radial and ulnar arteries, and median cubital vein.
- **Ulnar notch of the elbow** – This area is commonly referred to as the "funny bone" and contains the ulnar nerve.
- **Femoral triangle** – This area is bordered by the sartorius muscle, the adductor longus muscle, and the inguinal ligament and contains the femoral nerve, femoral artery, femoral vein, great saphenous vein, and lymph nodes.
- **Popliteal fossa** – The area on the posterior aspect of the knee bordered by the gastrocnemius muscle and the hamstrings and contains the tibial and common peroneal nerves, the popliteal artery, and popliteal vein.
- **Abdomen** – The upper area of the abdomen under the ribs. On the right side is the liver and gallbladder and on the left side is the spleen and aorta.
- **Upper lumbar area** – The area just inferior to the ribs and lateral to the spine where the kidneys are located should be massaged with caution. No heavy percussion.

Special Populations

CLIENTS WITH CANCER

When performing a massage, the client's well-being is of the utmost importance. As such, the therapist should be aware of the contraindications of performing massage on a cancer patient. A complete medical history should be taken, and the physician or oncologist should be consulted to determine if massage is a recommended and suitable form of treatment. Factors to consider are:

- Location and type of cancer
- Stage of the cancer
- Additional sites for metastasis
- Treatment level of the cancer
- Immune system condition of the person at the time of the massage
- Stamina level and attitude of the person

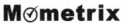

During the actual massage, light or moderate pressure should be used. Areas where tumors are known to exist should not be subjected to deep massage.

PREGNANT WOMEN

During a normal pregnancy, the mother can benefit from a massage, which will aid in decreasing the discomfort and aches associated with the back pain, leg pain, stress, and fatigue that occur during pregnancy. In order to provide the best care for the mother, it is important to note the mother's condition and to absolutely avoid massage when there is a risk of toxemia or pre-eclampsia. Massage is not an ideal way to address the high blood pressure, edema, nausea, and diarrhea associated with these conditions. Furthermore, massage can actually do harm to the mother. To prep the client, the massage therapist must ensure that both the mother and unborn child are in a comfortable position on the table, preferably facing up and in a semi-reclined position. If the client is lying on her side, it is important to place pillows under the head and between the knees to help support the back. Avoiding massage in the abdominal area is indicated. In addition, the therapist should not have the mother lie prone on her abdomen if she is in the latter stages of pregnancy.

BENEFITS

While pregnancy is generally considered a happy time in a woman's life, it can bring about many physical changes that cause additional strain and stress on the body. These physical changes include a shifting of the joints to accommodate weight gain and the stretching of the ligaments to prepare the body for delivery. Some of these changes are due to hormones, and they can cause a pregnant woman to feel additional strain, which can only be relieved through rest and relaxation. The areas that are most often subjected to stresses during pregnancy include the neck, back, hips, legs, and feet. During massage, supporting cushions and bolsters can increase the comfort level of the mother and allow her to fully enjoy the benefits of massage. These benefits include inducing a relaxed state, improving the body's circulation, and soothing the nerves. The most common positions for the mother during massage include lying in the side-lying position and, during the earliest parts of the pregnancy, lying in the prone position.

SPECIFIC PROCEDURES

It is advised that massage therapy be performed in the prone position only during the first trimester, before the new mother is "showing." Reducing the time spent in this position helps to keep the fetus safe. At no time should prenatal massage be performed on the abdominal area. If the mother indicates problems with nausea, vomiting, diarrhea, or unusual vaginal discharge, massage should be withheld until the physician has been notified. In addition, if there is high blood pressure, lack of fetal movement, severe edema, or any abdominal pain, the mother should be referred to her physician immediately, as these symptoms can indicate a severe condition like toxemia or pre-eclampsia. A less serious condition to be aware of during prenatal massage would be the presence of varicose veins. Light effleurage may be performed in these areas, but moderate to heavy massage techniques should be avoided.

INFANTS

There is no reason why infants cannot receive as many positive benefits from massage as adults. There are some special considerations, however, when administering massage treatments to an infant. The duration of an infant massage is typically shorter, usually lasting about 15 minutes. Because infants cannot express themselves verbally, the massage therapist needs to be especially sensitive to signs of discomfort. It is best to use natural oil for lubrication. An infant massage usually starts with a client in the supine position. While in this position, the face, torso, arms, legs, and feet can be massaged. Effleurage, petrissage, and tapotement can all be used during an infant

88

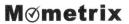

massage. After a while, the infant can be placed into the prone position so that the back and neck can be massaged.

ELDERLY CLIENTS

Elderly individuals can receive many benefits from massage. Their skin and bones, however, may be more sensitive to stress and strain, so the massage therapist needs to be especially gentle when dealing with an elderly client. Also, elderly clients are more likely to be modest, and may require more privacy when changing clothes. Elderly clients are likely to need special assistance mounting and dismounting the massage table. Massage is contraindicated in elderly individuals with varicose veins, blood clots, or bedsores. At times, the improved circulation generated by massage therapy can confuse or disorient elderly clients, so the massage therapist needs to be especially sensitive to any signs of distress.

DISABLED CLIENTS

Massage can be extremely beneficial for disabled individuals, so long as proper precautions are taken. Obviously, the precise precautions will depend on the disability. Individuals with sensory impairment, deafness or blindness for example, can receive normal massage therapy, though the therapist needs to be especially careful to clearly explain the success of the elements of the treatment. Clients who are on crutches are likely to have excessive strain on their triceps and wrists, while clients using wheelchairs are likely to have excessive tension in the muscles of the upper arm and back. When dealing with a paralyzed client, be sure to use gentle pressure, as the client will not be able to indicate injurious amounts of stress.

AMPUTEES

Loss of a limb can happen due to injury or accident, or due to an illness like cancer. Some amputees will have been fitted with a prosthetic limb. The client may be experiencing soreness at the attachment of the prosthesis or may have sore muscles from compensating and there could be postural deviations. There is great benefit to massage for amputees, but there are some considerations. The client may need assistance getting on to or off of the massage table. A client may or may not want to remove the prosthesis for the massage. The practitioner should always ask about the wishes of the client and ask if it is okay to massage at the prosthetic attachment. The client may also be experiencing phantom pain. Phantom pain is the sensation of having pain in a limb that is no longer there. Massaging the contralateral (opposite side) limb will sometimes help with phantom pain by causing a reflex effect. Be sure to check in with the client regarding pressure and any unpleasant effects that they may be experiencing from the massage. Bolsters should be used to provide the most comfortable position possible.

Classes of Medications

FAMILIARITY WITH BASIC PHARMACOLOGY

Pharmacology is the study of the effects that drugs have on living organisms. With a large number of individuals on prescription therapy, it may be common for the massage practitioner to encounter someone who is on drug therapy, but also needs the services of a massage therapist. Medications can cause side effects that, if not made known to the massage practitioner, will continue in spite of treatment. As an example, some medications cause muscle pain and weakness. When the therapist is knowledgeable about the types of medications a client is taking, he or she can then adapt the massage sessions to avoid certain areas. Additionally, some medications may provide the same benefits as those obtained by massage. In these cases, the individual may see a decreased need for medication due to the relief obtained through massage. Part of the initial consultation should

Pathology, Contraindications, Areas of Caution, and Special Populations

involve taking an inventory of the medications, supplements, vitamins, and herbs the client is taking.

ANTI-ANXIETY DRUGS

Anti-anxiety drugs influence the central nervous system and calm an individual's violent reaction to stress. There are two classes of anti-anxiety drugs:

- **Benzodiazepines** – act by reducing the activity of the neurons in the brain; common brands include Halcion, Valium, Xanax, and Ativan; during massage, client is at risk of entering a deep parasympathetic state, and should be monitored for dizziness
- **Buspirone HCl** – acts by reducing the uptake of dopamine and serotonin in the brain; sold under the brand name BuSpar; client should receive extra stimulation during massage, as the nervous system may be suppressed

ANTIDEPRESSANTS

Antidepressant medications alter the chemistry of the brain in order to alleviate the symptoms of depression. These drugs often take up to a month of use before yielding any positive results. There are three major classes of antidepressants, along with some other miscellaneous medications:

- **Tricyclics** – act by influencing the production of norepinephrine, serotonin, and acetylcholine; common brands include Tofranil, Elavil, and Norpramin; may result in dizziness during massage
- **Monoamine oxidase inhibitors** – act by limiting the activity of monoamine oxidase; common brands include Marplan and Nardate; sleepiness and dizziness may result from massage
- **Selective serotonin reuptake inhibitors** – act by managing the neurotransmitter serotonin; common brands include Prozac, Zoloft, Lexapro, Paxil, and Celexa; massage can occasionally lead to nausea or abdominal pain
- **Miscellaneous anti-depressants** – common brands include Effexor, Wellbutrin, and Serzone

ANTI-INFLAMMATORIES AND ANALGESICS

These medications are typically prescribed for individuals suffering from muscle pain. For this reason, massage therapists should be careful not to unwittingly injure a patient whose pain threshold is lower than normal. There are five classes of anti-inflammatories and analgesics:

- **Salicylates** – reduce fever and sensitivity to pain; common brands include Aspirin and Doan's Aspirin; vigorous massage should be avoided
- **Acetaminophen** – reduces pain and fever, but does not reduce inflammation; may be combined with caffeine or barbiturates; common brands include Tylenol and Anacin; massage should be gentle
- **Nonsteroidal anti-inflammatory drugs** – reduce inflammation and pain; common brands include Celebrex, Advil, Excedrin, Nuprin, and Aleve; watch out for abdominal bleeding and nausea
- **Steroidal anti-inflammatory drugs** – reduce inflammation, pain, and edema; common brands include Cortisone, Prednisol, and Decadron; deep-tissue massage should not be performed on clients who have been taking these drugs for a long time
- **Opioids, mixed opioids** – common brands include Codeine, OxyContin, Percocet, Darvon, Vicodin, and Demerol; morphine is also an opioid; massage should not include deep-tissue work, and the therapist should monitor the client's responsiveness

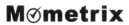

AUTONOMIC NERVOUS SYSTEM DISORDER MEDICATIONS

These drugs are designed to treat conditions affecting the sympathetic and parasympathetic nervous systems. There are four classes of autonomic nervous system disorder medications:

- **Cholinergics** – act in a manner similar to the parasympathetic nervous system; common brands include Urecholine and Carbastat; massage should be gentle and the client should be monitored for responsiveness
- **Anticholinergics** – these drugs either stimulate or suppress particular organs or parts of the nervous system; common brands include Atropine, Ditropan, and Anaspaz; massage should be performed with the particular action of the drug taken into consideration
- **Adrenergic drugs** – act by stimulating the sympathetic nervous system; common brands include Dopamine, Epinephrine, and Albuterol; it may take longer to induce a parasympathetic response from a client taking this kind of medication
- **Adrenergic blockers** – hinder the action of the sympathetic nervous system; common brands include Flomax, Migranal, and Cardura; it will be easy for the client to enter a deep parasympathetic state

CARDIOVASCULAR DRUGS

Cardiovascular drugs either expand blood vessels or decrease the response of the sympathetic nervous system, thereby reducing the amount of stress placed on the heart. There are seven major classes of cardiovascular drugs:

- **Beta blockers** – act by reducing the impact of the sympathetic nervous system on the heart; common brands include Inderal, Normodyne, and Levatol; blood pressure should be monitored during massage
- **Calcium channel blockers** – expand the blood vessels; common brands include Norvasc, Cardene, and Isoptin; clients may suffer from dizziness, low blood pressure, and flushing
- **ACE inhibitors** – increase evacuation of water and sodium; common brands include Lotensin, Captopril, and Vasotec; may result in extremely low blood pressure
- **Digitalis** – strengthens and improves the efficiency of the heart; common brands include Digitek and Lanoxin; circulatory massage should be avoided
- **Antilipemic drugs** – reduce the amount of cholesterol in the blood; common brands include Questran, Lopid, Zocor, and Crestor; constipation and cramping are two common concerns that should be considered before the initiation of massage therapy
- **Diuretics** – increases the amount of urine created by the kidneys; common brands include Lasix, Bumex, Thalitone, and Lozol; care should be taken to avoid stressing the kidneys or reducing the blood pressure to a dangerous level
- **Antianginal medications** – either increase the amount of oxygen sent to the heart or reduce the heart's need for oxygen; common brands include Cedocard, Monoket, Nitrostat, and Nitro-Glycerin; the massage should be stopped immediately if hypotension, dizziness, or cramping occur

CANCER DRUGS

Cancer drugs are administered to kill or stop the production of cancer cells. Remember that these drugs act by more or less attacking all the cells of the body, and clients will therefore be severely debilitated. For this reason, extreme care should be taken during massage therapy. There are six major classes of cancer drugs:

- **Alkylating drugs** – common types include nitrogen mustards, ethylamines, alkyl sulfonates, triazenes, piperazines, and nitrosoureas
- **Antimetabolite drugs** – common brands include Cladribine, Aminopterin, and Cytarabine
- **Antineoplastics** – can be antibiotic, hormonal, natural, or other; these drugs inhibit the growth and development of malignant cells

CLOT MANAGEMENT DRUGS

Clot management drugs manage the body's ability to stop bleeding. In a normal body, blood clots are formed from a combination of red blood cells, white blood cells, and platelets. There are two classes of clot management drugs:

- **Anticoagulants** – encourage the liver to produce chemicals that limit the formation of new blood clots; common brands include Heparin and Lovenox; clients on this medication may be susceptible to bruising
- **Antiplatelet drugs** – act by preventing platelets in the blood from congregating at potential clot sites; common brands include Aspirin, Pletal, and Empirin; clients may be especially susceptible to bruising

DIABETES MANAGEMENT DRUGS

The number of people taking diabetes management medications is steadily increasing in the United States. A massage therapist must monitor the client closely during massage, as a sudden decrease in blood glucose levels has the potential to induce a hypoglycemic episode. There are two classes of diabetes management drugs:

- **Insulin** – enables the body to obtain energy from glucose in the blood; common brands include Humulin, Lantus, and Novolin; the injection area should be avoided during massage, and, if possible, clients should receive massage towards the beginning of their insulin cycle
- **Oral glucose management drugs** – reduce the production of sugar in the liver and increase the production of insulin in the pancreas; common brands include Diabinese, Glucotrol, lucophage, and Precose; clients are at an increased risk of experiencing a hypoglycemic episode when taking this kind of medication

MUSCLE RELAXANTS

Muscle relaxants reduce the amount of tension in muscular tissue. For this reason, it is especially important for massage therapists to be restrained in the amount of force they use during bodywork. These drugs are primarily prescribed to alleviate muscle spasms and the resulting pain. There are two classes of muscle relaxants:

- **Centrally-acting skeletal muscle relaxants** – act by depressing the central nervous system; common brands include Soma, Paraflex, Valium, Norflex, and Flexeril.
- **Peripherally-acting skeletal muscle relaxants** – act by diminishing the contractions of the muscles; commonly sold under the brand name Dantrium; stretching should not exceed the client's normal range of motion during massage.

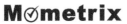

THYROID SUPPLEMENT DRUGS

Thyroid supplement medications are prescribed to treat hypothyroidism. There are three classes of thyroid supplement drugs:

- **Levothyroxine sodium** – imitate the natural secretions of the thyroid; common brands include Synthroid, Eltroxin, and Levoxyl; massage is indicated, and should not react with medications in any adverse way
- **Desiccated extract** – imitate the actions of the hormones produced by a healthy thyroid; common brands include Armour Thyroid, Nature-Thyroid, and Westhroid; no real effect on massage
- **Liothyronine sodium** – these drugs fulfill the same functions as other thyroid supplements, and are generally only prescribed when the others are ineffective; common brands include Cytomel and Triostat; no negative interaction with massage

DRUG

Drugs are any chemical or herbal substances that are used to relieve the symptoms of an illness or disease. The term "drug" can also be used to refer to illegal substances that alter the mind's perception and the body's movement. Oftentimes, the drugs prescribed by a physician can produce adverse side effects on the human body that can interfere with any benefits obtained the drug. Some drugs have the ability to affect an entire system of the body, including drugs that affect the circulatory system. Some other drugs cause only a localized reaction, such as those used to alleviate the pain of a broken leg.

PROCEDURE FOR CLASSIFYING DRUGS

The federal Food and Drug Administration classifies drugs in order to protect the safety of the consumer. Drugs do not affect all individuals in the same manner, as a person's age, body weight, and height help to determine how fast the body absorbs the drug. Drugs are given a generic name when they are created by a pharmaceutical company. A specific trade name is then given to help consumers identify it and make it easier to remember. Drugs are classified according to their therapeutic abilities; thus, the same drug can fall under more than one classification.

HERBAL SUPPLEMENTS AND VITAMINS

Herbal remedies have been around for many years, and their origins can be traced back to many cultural groups, including Native American and Chinese societies. Herbs have many uses, from cooking, to decoration, to healing. Depending on the purpose of the plant and the need for it, all parts may be used, from the flowers and seeds down to the roots. Compared to chemically-based drugs, herbs are more commonly prescribed by physicians in other parts of the world. Approximately 25% of all prescription drugs come from a natural botanical source, unlike other drugs that are chemically manufactured in a lab environment. People tend to purchase herbs and supplements as a means of preventing disease and maintaining good health, and as an additional form of treatment that is used in conjunction with standard pharmaceutical treatment methods. The massage therapist should have an understanding of the effects of herbal supplements because of their widespread use, and also because their effects could interact with prescription medications.

OPIOID AND NON-OPIOID ANALGESICS

Opioid analgesics are considered a narcotic while non-opioid analgesics are not. Opioid analgesics work on opioid receptors which are present throughout the nervous system and are involved in the control and signaling of pain. Non-opioid analgesics do not work on the central nervous system and instead directly affect the injured body tissues. Opioids will decrease the body's awareness of the pain while non-opioids will affect chemical changes that are occurring at the site of injury. This will

Pathology, Contraindications, Areas of Caution, and Special Populations

decrease inflammation and pain. Opioid analgesics do not have an anti-inflammatory effect on the body. One big difference between the two analgesics is that non-opioid analgesics do not create dependence and addiction in the way that opioids do. Withdrawal symptoms will be felt with the long-term use of opioids which is not seen in non-opioid analgesics. When opioid analgesics are lowered in dose or discontinued, the body will develop withdrawal symptoms. This makes it more difficult for someone to stop treatment with opioids and can lead to addiction. Both types have side effects. Non-opioids can cause renal toxicity and gastric irritation and bleeding with long term use. Opioids can depress respiration, cause sedation, and constipation.

Benefits and Physiological Effects of Techniques that Manipulate Soft Tissue

Identification of the Physiological Effects of Soft Tissue Manipulation

PHYSIOLOGICAL EFFECTS OF MASSAGE

Western massage, otherwise known as Swedish massage, helps to relax the body, increase metabolism, speed healing, and provide emotional and physical relaxation. Similar massages on two individuals can produce two entirely different reactions. Techniques used in Swedish massage include light touches and gentle stimulation over the skin, which produce reflexive sensations. Mechanically stimulating the body by increasing pressure on the muscles and tissues results in an increase in blood flow to the area, causing an increase in nutrients and oxygen as well as the removal of wastes from the muscle. By the end of the massage session, the body is in a more relaxed state. There is an increase in flexibility and a decrease in pain. An increase in the production of sweat and oil from the glands can be seen by the end of the massage. There is an improvement in blood flow to the area, resulting in a temporary color change in the skin. Finally, the temperature of the skin increases.

EFFECTS OF MASSAGE ON THE MUSCULAR STRUCTURE

When a massage is being performed, the muscles undergo a transformation that helps them increase their nutritional intake, improves circulation, and helps to stimulate cellular activity within the muscle. Massage relaxes tense muscles and helps to alleviate the pain associated with muscle spasms. During a massage, blood passes through the muscular tissue at a rate that is three times greater than when the muscle is at rest. This action brings new supplies of blood to the area, and assists with the removal of waste material. After strenuous exercise, massage helps to alleviate the pain, stiffness, and soreness associated with the exercise. If massage is prescribed as a therapy after an injury, there is less scarring and buildup of connective tissue in the muscles. Range of motion is also increased through massage. Circulation is also increased, which helps to reduce the time lost due to the injury.

EFFECTS OF MASSAGE ON THE NERVOUS SYSTEM

The nervous system is comprised of the central nervous system (made up of the brain and spinal cord) and the peripheral nervous system (made up of the autonomic nervous system, cranial nerves, and spinal nerves). The nervous system has the ability to be either stimulated or soothed, depending on the type of muscle massage being utilized. Techniques that stimulate the body include friction, percussion, and vibration. Light rubbing, rolling or wringing of the skin is known as the technique of friction. Percussion involves a series of tapping to increase the nervous irritability. Depending on the duration, percussion has the ability to numb the nerves within the area. Vibration involves applying shaking or trembling movements on the body part. The end result is the stimulation of peripheral nerves. Soothing techniques that produce a calming effect include light stroking of the skin and pétrissage, which are light, kneading movements on the skin. Putting pressure on a specific trigger point desensitizes the area and releases hypertension in the muscle.

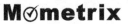

EFFECTS OF MASSAGE ON AUTONOMIC NERVOUS SYSTEM

The autonomic nervous system is divided into two distinct areas: the sympathetic nervous system and the parasympathetic nervous system. The sympathetic nervous system is responsible for the "fight or flight" response, while the parasympathetic system counters these effects and helps to return the body to a relaxed state by reducing the heart rate and increasing circulation to bring about a relaxed state of being. The sympathetic nervous system, by contrast, increases the alertness of the body through the release of adrenaline and epinephrine. When a massage is performed, the reaction from the autonomic nervous system is initially one of invigoration, which gradually mellows into relaxation and sedation. The parasympathetic nervous system is stimulated, leading to a reduction in epinephrine, norepinephrine, and blood pressure.

EFFECTS OF MASSAGE ON CIRCULATORY SYSTEM

When techniques such as massage, pressure, stroking, and percussion are performed on the body, the circulatory system responds in a favorable manner, which benefits the entire body. Stroking the skin lightly causes dilation in the capillaries. Applying stronger pressure while stroking leads to the skin taking on a flushed look and a longer-lasting period of dilation. Percussion of the muscles causes the blood vessels to contract; they gradually ease up and cause a relaxed state. Applying friction to the muscles and skin rapidly produces a response, in this case the flow of blood through the veins. It also accounts for the flow of interstitial fluid, which leads to a healthy cellular environment. Kneading the muscles causes the blood to flow into the deeper sections of arteries and veins. Lighter massage techniques are responsible for lymph circulation, as they diminish the tendency towards edema in these areas. Compression causes muscles to store a larger quantity of blood. Finally, all massage techniques should be directed towards the heart: from the ends of the appendages towards the torso and also from the head downward.

PAIN

ASSISTING WITH THE HEALING OF THE BODY AS A RESULT OF PAIN

The massage therapist should pay close attention to areas of concern in the patient's body before, during, and after the massage. Techniques used during the massage have the ability to alleviate any suffering caused by pain or stress. Of particular interest to the therapist are methods that can relieve the pain of a pain-spasm-pain cycle, which is indicated by ischemia (decreased blood flow to the area within a muscle). A proper therapeutic massage increases blood flow to an area, creating pleasurable sensations where there was previously only marked pain. The nerve endings carry these signals to the brain, causing the overall feeling of calmness and relaxation throughout the body. To combat ischemia, the massage therapist should focus on breaking the pain-spasm-pain cycle and increasing mobility in that area. Through therapeutic palpations, the exact area of pain can be identified. The therapist can then focus the massage in that area, reduce the amount of lactic acid within the muscle, and introduce oxygen and other nutrients to help speed healing.

MANAGEMENT OF PAIN

Pain management is one of the benefits obtained through massage therapy, as the muscle receives an influx of blood circulating through the tissue. Through a process known as gate control theory, the transmission of pain sensations from the affected area is interrupted and prevented from reaching the central nervous system. This is accomplished through stimulating the cutaneous receptors. Massage techniques such as rubbing and applying pressure also prevent the pain sensation from reaching the receptors in the brain. An example of this response is the reduction in the degree of pain that results from rubbing an area that has been struck.

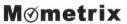

ALLEVIATING STRESS

When a person experiences significant stress in his or her life, it causes physiological and psychological changes in the body. At the physiological level, heart rates can increase, adrenaline rises, sweating may occur, and tightness can be felt within the muscles of the body as the skin prepares for a "fight or flight" response. Psychologically, a person may feel overwhelmed, depressed, moody, or sad, and may even take drastic measures to deal with the stress, such as consuming alcohol or using drugs. Massage is indicated as a means to help alleviate negative stress through the personal human contact inherent in treatment, and through ridding the body of toxins and waste in the cells. During the initial massage therapy consultation, the practitioner should be aware of any indicators of extreme stress and outline a plan that will bring relaxation to the client in a timely manner. At no point should the practitioner assume the role of a psychotherapist or counselor.

PAIN VS. STRESS

Pain causes sensations that range from slight to severe. It indicates potential damage to the tissues or possible destruction within the body. Pain can be an indication of damage to nerve endings that lie beneath the surface of the skin, damage to the periosteum of the bones, damage to blood vessels and arteries, and finally, deeper damage to internal organs and muscles. The body's response to pain is both physical and physiological, which means that the body's response to pain mimics the reaction that the body has to stress. Stress is any condition that causes strain on the body or tension within the body. It can affect the internal balance and harmony within the body. Stress affects each person differently at varying levels. Overall, increased stress can be detrimental to the health of the individual. The body's reactions to stress include an increased heart rate, the secretion of "fight or flight" hormones from the adrenal gland, deeper breathing, and increased blood pressure.

DOPAMINE AND SEROTONIN

During a massage, some of the chemicals released within the body produce positive physiological effects. Neurotransmitters such as dopamine and serotonin are released, which contribute to pain control and mood elevation. One neurotransmitter is dopamine, which helps to control the brain's emotions, motor skills, and feelings of pleasure or pain. Serotonin is another type of neurotransmitter that also helps regulate moods, behavior, appetite, and memory. Low levels of serotonin can contribute to depression, anxiety, sleep disorders, and even personality disorders. Massage helps to increase the levels of these neurotransmitters within the body, and leads to a sense of peacefulness and calmness that can help reduce stress. Massage also contributes to appetite control and increased functioning of the immune system.

CORRELATION BETWEEN THERAPEUTIC MASSAGE AND ANATOMY AND PHYSIOLOGY

Therapeutic massage is defined as the process of applying techniques such as effleurage, pétrissage, stretching, and stroking on the muscular structure of the body to ease pains in the tendons, ligaments, muscles, and surface of the skin. This type of massage is intended to create a sense of calmness and relaxation, as well as to alleviate any pain, stiffness, or soreness in the body. Increased circulation, greater flexibility, improved muscle tone, and improved posture are additional effects that therapeutic massage has on the body. Having a basic understanding of human anatomy allows the massage therapist to focus on the parts of the body that require additional consideration, and also enables him to avoid measures which can cause pain to the client. Physiological changes include the lowering of the client's blood pressure, reduction in the heart rate, and slower, deeper breathing, all of which contribute to the relaxed state of the client.

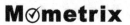

Psychological Aspects and Benefits of Touch

EFFECTS OF MASSAGE ON PRODUCTION OF SEROTONIN AND DOPAMINE

Dopamine and serotonin are neurotransmitters. Dopamine affects brain functions involved in fine movement, emotional response, and the ability to experience pleasure and pain. Increased dopamine levels lead to improvement in mood, alertness, and sex drive. Low dopamine levels interfere with cognition and movement. Parkinson's disease is caused by an inability to produce dopamine. Serotonin is synthesized in the brain and is found in the blood stream, brain, and intestinal walls. It has many effects on the body including behavior, appetite, blood pressure, temperature regulation, memory, and learning ability. Higher levels of serotonin seem to increase feelings of calm and well-being. Lower levels of serotonin can cause depression, eating disorders, personality disorders, sleep disturbances, and schizophrenia. Serotonin helps to counterbalance the negative effects that stress has on the body. Massage increases both the levels of dopamine and serotonin in the body. This leads to decreased stress and depression and an elevation of mood. Though the exact reason as to why serotonin and dopamine increase with massage is not known, it is believed that the relaxation response and the decrease in cortisol are factors that contribute to their increase.

BENEFITS OF MASSAGE FOR THOSE WITH BODY ISSUES

Research has proven that massage is an effective tool for helping to increase self-image and self-worth in those who are struggling with self-esteem and addiction issues. Massage has been shown to increase awareness of the body and allow the recipient to relax. Touch in a therapeutic, non-threatening environment can help someone suffering from body issues become more accepting of their body. Massage research involving women with eating disorders has shown that, after receiving regular massage, the women reported decreases in body dissatisfaction and an increase in dopamine and serotonin levels, which increase mood and regulate appetite. A massage practitioner working with a client who has body issues must be sure to use extra care and compassion to make the client as comfortable and confident as possible. Regular massage can allow someone with body issues to learn to develop a healthy connection to their body, build self-esteem, and encourage good health practices.

EMOTIONAL RELEASE

It is not uncommon for a client to experience an emotional release while receiving a massage. This can be due to chemical and structural changes occurring in the tissue that cause emotions to be released and brought to the recipient's attention. The release can happen for many reasons, and all emotional releases should be treated with calmness and respect for the client. The practitioner must maintain personal boundaries at all times. The first step is to acknowledge the emotional release and allow the client to feel supported and safe. Do not remove physical contact unless the client has asked for touch to cease. Have the client take deep breaths and ask if the massage should be continued. If the client would like to be left alone, the practitioner may leave the room if the client is safe. If the client would like to continue the massage, the practitioner may continue as normal. It is important to remember that massage practitioners are not mental health therapists and should not attempt to counsel a client. Allowing a client to talk about the release during the massage is acceptable. Offering a referral to a mental health professional is advised if the practitioner feels it necessary.

PAIN GATE CONTROL THEORY

The nervous system contains various types of receptors that register sensations and transmit those sensations to the brain via the spinal cord. Nociceptors are the type of receptor that transmits pain signals. There are also thermoreceptors for registering temperature and mechanoreceptors which respond to any mechanical stimulation including pressure, stretching, touch, or vibration. The pain gate control theory explains how pain sensations can be disrupted by massage. Nociceptors send their pain signals through both large- and small-diameter nerve fibers. Other receptors, like mechanoreceptors or thermoreceptors, send their signals through large-diameter nerve fibers. When the mechanoreceptors and thermoreceptors are stimulated through massage, their sensations travel along these larger diameter nerve fibers and suppress the pain sensations before they enter the spinal column. The gate is essentially closed on the pain sensations because there is not enough fiber width to send the signal and the pain is diminished. This example can be easily demonstrated by applying ice or rubbing an injury immediately after it happens. The sensations of cold or mechanical force to the tissue are transmitted to the brain but the pain sensations diminish.

NEGATIVE EFFECTS OF STRESS ON THE BODY

Any condition or situation, whether physical or psychological, that causes tension or strain qualifies as stress. What is stressful for one person may not be to another. However, the physiological effects of stress are the same in everybody. The adrenal glands become active under stress and release the hormones adrenaline and cortisol. These are meant to give a boost both mentally and physically and to sharpen the senses in times of danger. Working with the pituitary and the hypothalamus, these hormones can increase muscle tone and blood pressure and deepen inhalation. The blood flow will be directed away from digestion and sent to the muscles to prepare for action. The body prepares to break down proteins to form glucose, the kidneys retain fluid, and red blood cells are mobilized. This is all necessary in a state of emergency. The problem is that many people live in this constant state of stress and eventually it leads to illness and disease. Sustained levels of stress hormones can cause ulcers, high blood pressure, a depressed immune system, and atherosclerosis. The effect of constant high levels of cortisol in the blood can also slow the body's healing process and the ability to fight infections.

Benefits of Soft Tissue Manipulation for Specific Client Populations

BENEFITS OF MASSAGE IN PREGNANCY

Massage during pregnancy can be very beneficial. Studies have shown prenatal massage to be effective for relief of the anxiety and depression that some women experience during pregnancy. It is also helpful for relieving the joint and muscle aches that are common. Weight gain and softening of ligaments to prepare for delivery can cause discomfort and massage can offer excellent relief. Massage will also decrease the level of stress, which has been shown to decrease complications during birth and even protect the baby against such complications as low birth weight. A mother who is healthier and more relaxed during pregnancy will generally give birth to a healthier and more relaxed baby. Massage will also decrease the edema or swelling that is common during pregnancy and can improve the sciatic nerve pain that many women experience. Back and neck pain and tension, as well as headaches, decrease with massage during pregnancy and women often report better sleep after receiving massage. The soft tissues and muscles become more oxygenated and the overall sense of well-being improves, which makes for a better and more comfortable pregnancy.

BENEFITS OF MASSAGE ON THE ELDERLY

The following are benefits of massage on the elderly:

- Massage can alleviate or offer relief from age-related discomforts such as painful joints, muscle weakness and pain, and decreased mobility.
- Massage can assist with increasing the immune response to prevent illnesses.

- Massage may have an effect on slowing the aging process.
- Massage can help increase mobility, improve strength, and increase flexibility, counteracting deficits that occur due to the aging process and decreased activity.
- Activities of daily living can become easier with regular massage. Such things as climbing stairs, cooking, dressing, and bathing will see improvement with the increase in strength and mobility received from massage.
- Abdominal massage can improve digestion and decrease constipation, which is common in the elderly.
- Massage can relieve anxiety and depression for the elderly, the same as with younger adults.
- Regular massage can provide a social connection for someone who may not have friends and family to spend time with.

BENEFITS FOR CLIENTS UNDERGOING CANCER TREATMENT

There has been much debate over whether massage is appropriate for those diagnosed with cancer. Through research, however, it has been discovered that, with an educated practitioner and certain precautions, massage can be very beneficial to cancer patients. The greatest benefits are the relief or control of pain and relief from depression. It has also proven effective in preventing nausea, relieving insomnia, increasing feelings of relaxation, reducing anxiety, and helping to restore a body image that may be damaged due to treatments. Clients with cancer will also see a decrease in muscle tension, spasms, and fatigue. Digestion and elimination will improve with massage, and edema and swelling will decrease. Overall, the client with cancer who receives regular massage will generally see an improved and more positive outlook and feelings of improved self-esteem. Studies have also shown that massage increases certain immune factors in the blood. Before massaging a client with cancer, it is important for a massage practitioner to understand all of the factors involved with the individual case, and it is best to consult the client's physician for specific precautions.

BENEFITS FOR THE CRITICALLY ILL

Massage to the critically ill is mostly delivered with the intent to provide a gentle and compassionate form of touch therapy which will give comfort and relaxation during a difficult time. The primary benefits of massage in this situation are to control discomfort and pain and improve mobility. Often, patients who are critically ill will be disoriented. Massage can help to reduce confusion and bring the patient back to a more centered self-awareness. Someone who is critically ill may live with feelings of isolation or fear. Compassionate touch can make them feel cared for and reduce those feelings. Patients who are critically ill may not be receiving comforting touch because loved ones may fear hurting them, so touch therapy is valuable in providing the human connection that may be missing. Massage can also help the patient to develop a more positive attitude and outlook on their illness and bring a better sense of well-being in general.

Soft Tissue Techniques

BASIC MASSAGE MOVEMENTS

The basic massage movements are as follows:

- **Touch** – includes superficial and deep massage
- **Gliding or effleurage movements** – moving the hand or forearm over the body while applying varying amounts of pressure; can be aura stroking, superficial, or deep
- **Kneading** – includes pétrissage, rolling, lifting, and squeezing of the skin

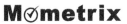

- **Friction** – causing one layer of skin tissue to rub against another; can be performed by rolling, compressing, wringing, and vibrating
- **Percussion** – alternately striking the surface of the skin through cupping, slapping, tapping, and beating
- **Joint movements** – manipulating the limbs of the body through passive or active movements

TOUCH

Touch is defined as the action of initiating skin-to-skin contact between the massage therapist's hand and the client's body. Touch does not involve any movement. The pressure can range from extremely light to deep pressure, depending on the type of reaction the therapist is trying to achieve. Touch can have a calming physiological effect on the client. The massage therapist should open the massage session with a few moments of touch as a means of connecting with the client and becoming comfortable with his personal body space. This gentle touching is also performed at the end of the massage to signal the end of the session and provide a sense of closure for both the client and the therapist. Deep pressure can also be applied through touch. In this sense, touch is applied to calm, anesthetize, or stimulate the muscles. It is often used to soothe muscle spasms or alleviate pain. Force is applied through body movements rather than by relying only upon the strength of the therapist's arms.

GLIDING TECHNIQUES
ETHEREAL STROKING AND FEATHER STROKING

The types of movements that are based on maneuvering the hand over the client's body with varying degrees of pressure are known as gliding techniques. Ethereal or aura stroking is the process in which the practitioner glides his hands over the length of the client's body, but does not actually touch the body. The intention of this practice, according to some philosophies, is to smooth over the energy field that surrounds the body. A second type of gliding technique is feather stroking, which involves making long, gentle strokes from the center of the body outward.

EFFLEURAGE AND DEEP GLIDING

Effleurage is a common Swedish massage technique that calls for successive strokes over a long surface of the body. The pressure is increased with each stroke. Superficial gliding involves applying light pressure to the body with the hand over all surfaces. This gives the therapist a chance to assess the condition of the muscles prior to commencing the massage. The amount of pressure exerted, the part of the hand that is used, and the way that the pressure is applied must all be considered when the deep gliding technique is being performed. Deep gliding strokes are designed to stretch and broaden the muscle tissue and fascia. It is best to make these movements towards the heart to encourage blood and lymph flow.

PÉTRISSAGE

Kneading, or pétrissage, is used on the fleshy parts of the body to bring about movement of fluid in deep tissues and help stretch the muscle tissue. The skin is generally raised between the hands and kneaded with firm pressure in circular motions. Often, both hands are used to perform this motion. In the type of pétrissage known as fulling, the tissue is lifted up and then spread out to enhance the area in between the muscular tissue. Another form of pétrissage is called skin rolling. In this method, the fingers pick up the skin in alternate motions and gently pull it away from the underlying tissues to create a stretching of the fascia. This motion warms the skin and helps to remove any buildup of adhesions on the tissue.

FRICTION

Friction helps to move the superficial layers of tissue against the deeper tissues within the body. The action of applying friction creates warmth when the therapist presses tissue upon tissue, thereby flattening it, releasing fluids from the tissue, and also stretching it at the same time. The warmth produced also causes the client's metabolic rate to increase.

CIRCULAR AND CROSS-FIBER FRICTION

Types of friction methods include circular friction and cross-fiber friction. As the name implies, circular friction involves moving the fingers or hands over the client's skin in a circular pattern. Cross-fiber friction is performed in a sharp, transverse direction to the muscle being worked on. This is the preferred method used when a specific muscle group is being rehabilitated; it promotes the rebuilding of elastic tissue fibers.

COMPRESSION, ROLLING, CHUCKING, WRINGING, AND VIBRATION

The friction techniques of compression, rolling, chucking, wringing, and vibration that are used in massage are described below:

- **Compression** is the rhythmic movement of the hands or fingers on the muscular tissue. Palmar compression is directed onto the muscles, transverse from the bone. It does not require the use of oils or lotions and, in fact, can be performed over clothing. It is commonly used in sports massage.
- **Rolling** is the method in which a body part is rapidly passed back and forth between the hands. This results in warmth and encourages relaxation of the deeper muscle tissue.
- **Chucking** is the process by which the tissue is grabbed between the hands and moved up and down along the length of the bone. This method is performed rather quickly.
- **Wringing** is a process that is similar to wringing water from a towel. The hands move in opposing directions as the flesh is twisted against the bone.
- **Vibration** is a movement that is performed either manually or in conjunction with a device that produces continuous trembling movements against the muscle. This action helps to desensitize and numb the area.

PERCUSSION TECHNIQUES

Percussion movements are quick, striking motions that are made alternately against the body. This technique serves to stimulate the body. The movements do not involve the application of great force. The types of percussion movements are slapping, tapping, cupping, hacking, and beating.

SLAPPING AND TAPPING

Slapping involves applying pressure from the flat palm of the hand against the surface of the body. Tapping involves using the fingertips in such a way that only the pads of the fingers come in contact with the body. The fingers can be either held in a flexed position or straight. Either way, the pressure applied is very light.

CUPPING, HACKING, AND BEATING

Cupping involves shaping the hand into a curved shape prior to applying it to the body. This method is generally used on the rib area, and is a technique commonly used by respiratory therapists to eliminate buildup and congestion in the lungs. Hacking is the use of the ulnar side of the hands to strike the body, which causes an improvement in circulation and relaxation. Beating involves using loose fists to gently pound the body, and is considered the heaviest and deepest form of percussion. This technique is used primarily on the dense muscle tissues.

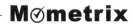

PASSIVE JOINT MOVEMENT

One type of joint movement is known as passive joint movement. It is generally performed when the client is in a relaxed state and the therapist is able to maneuver, exercise, and stretch a part of the body. PJM is also used to determine the extent of any injuries to the client, and to determine the exact range of motion that part of the body can achieve. Working the muscle and joint in this way allows the therapist to help improve the mobility of the joint and extend its range of motion. To perform the passive joint movement, the therapist must take care to move the limb only in the direction that it is designed to move, without any forceful or sharp gestures. If the movement is being done to assess damage, stopping at the point of the client's pain is indicated. To rehabilitate the joint, further extension of the limb is recommended.

ACTIVE JOINT MOVEMENT

In active joint movement, the client is responsible for contracting the muscle to perform the required movement of the joint. It is commonly used as an assessment tool to determine the exact capabilities and the range of motion of the client. The results can be benchmarked at the start of treatment, with a comparison made at the end of treatment to note the progress made. Active assistive joint movement is performed when the client attempts to move the joint through a series of movements. The therapist assists when the client no longer has the strength or ability to move the injured limb further. This is primarily a therapeutic device designed to restore mobility in the limb. Another type of joint movement is active resistive joint movement. In this action, the therapist or practitioner applies resistive force against the motion of the limb. This allows for the buildup of muscle strength that, in turn, leads to increased use of the limb. Resistive motions such as these can be applied to any body part.

End Feel, Hard End Feel, Soft End Feel, AND Empty End Feel

End feel, hard end feel, soft end feel, and empty end feel are defined below:

- **End feel** – This occurs when the practitioner moves a client's joint through the range of motion and, just before the end point, feels a change in the quality of the movement. This sense of resistance, whether attributable to physiologic or anatomic factors, is known as the end feel.
- **Hard end feel** – This is the feeling of bone rubbing against bone. A common location where this occurs is in the elbow joint.
- **Soft end feel** – This is the limitation that occurs when moving a joint due to the location of soft tissue, which prevents additional movement.
- **Empty end feel** – This is the presence of pain when moving a joint, which ends up causing restrictions on the full range of motion.

MYOFASCIAL RELEASE MASSAGE

Myofascial release massage's primary goal is to improve the condition and function of the fascial system and remove the constrictions caused by tight fascia. Restrictions in the fascia can cause nerves and blood and lymph vessels to become compressed and confined so its release will improve circulation and lymph flow. Myofascial release techniques will work both the superficial and the deep fascia. Superficial fascia consists of loose connective tissue and deep fascia is made up of dense connective tissue. The superficial fascia is found throughout the entire body just below the surface of the skin. It connects the skin to the deeper fascia. The deeper fascia surrounds and penetrates the muscles. Muscle tissue is inseparable from fascia. Myofascial release techniques will release the superficial fascia then connect to the deeper fascia to cause a release within the deeper level. This work will break up fibrous adhesions that have developed in the fascia, causing restriction, and will allow the tissues to more easily glide as they move against each other.

SKIN ROLLING

Skin rolling can be used to both assess the quality and condition of the skin and to release and loosen constricted tissue. To perform skin rolling, the practitioner picks up the skin and superficial fascia between the thumb and fingers. The skin is then rolled as more tissue is gathered and then slips out from under the thumbs. The move should be a smooth and continuous motion. The hands should be held close together and work in unison, pulling the superficial tissue away from the deeper tissue. The stroke should be done slowly and allow the tissue to release. The technique is most often performed on the back, but can be done on almost any body part. Skin rolling will warm and stretch the tissues and separate adhesions among the fascial sheaths. No lubricant should be used for this technique.

J-STROKE

The J-Stroke is a myofascial release stroke that is used to stretch and elongate contracted muscles and separate and align constricted fascia. It is usually applied with the thumbs but can be performed with the fingertips. It is applied as a friction stroke, moving the superficial tissues over the deeper layers. Start by making light contact with the skin using the thumb. The skin is then pulled back slightly from the direction the stroke is intended to move. Move deeper into the tissue to reach the fibrous tissue beneath. The thumb then hooks and rotates deeply into the tissue in the intended direction of the stroke. The line of the stroke generally follows the direction of the fibers of the underlying tissues. The stroke should continue as long as the superficial tissue allows. There should be no gliding of the thumb across the skin. It should be repeated three to five times on the same spot before moving backward and continuing to repeat the stroke.

CRANIOSACRAL PULSE

The craniosacral system is a system within the body that consists of the meninges, the cerebrospinal fluid that surrounds and protects the brain and spinal cord, and related bones and structures that control the input and outflow of fluid. This system is considered a hydraulic system with fluids in constant flow. The craniosacral pulse is the rhythmic flow of cerebrospinal fluid that is occurring within the craniosacral system. A trained practitioner can theoretically feel this pulse using a light touch at locations where the craniosacral membrane is attached to bone. The locations include the skull, the sacrum, and the tailbone. With practice, the craniosacral pulse can be differentiated from the cardiovascular pulse. The craniosacral pulse occurs in waves at a rate of about six to twelve cycles per minute. The waves consist of both a flexion and extension phase. The flexion phase is felt as a widening and front-to-back shortening of the skull. The extension phase is felt as a narrowing and front-to-back lengthening of the skull. It is most easily felt at the ankles, thighs, pelvis, thorax, and head.

CRANIOSACRAL THERAPY AND STILL POINT

Craniosacral therapy is designed to be a non-invasive, indirect, and gentle way to remove restrictive barriers and allow the craniosacral motion to be smooth and symmetrical. A trained practitioner will be able to feel abnormal motion and apply indirect techniques that will allow the craniosacral motion to be free of restriction. The techniques encourage movement that is away from the restriction and toward ease by having the practitioner follow the movement in the direction that is the most free. As the movement reaches its end point, the practitioner will hold immobile and allow the craniosacral flow to continue its cycle. As it continues its movement, the motion will move further into the direction of ease and the practitioner will take up the slack and hold. The tissue should be held at the farthest point of the cycle. This is repeated until the craniosacral system becomes quiet and still. This is known as the still point. Once the still point has been reached, the

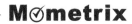

practitioner then releases the hold and feels the motion once again. At this point the system should move in a more symmetrical and easy manner with less or no restriction.

WORKING FROM GENERAL TO SPECIFIC THEN BACK TO GENERAL AGAIN WHEN APPLYING MASSAGE STROKES

Applying massage techniques from general to specific then back to general again is considered the general rule of massage. This rule is important because it allows the practitioner to prepare the area for more specific work by increasing blood flow and relaxing the tissues. General work will also allow the practitioner to palpate for areas in the tissue which may need more specific work. Working directly into a specific area may cause protective spasm by the surrounding tissues because it has not been prepared for deeper, more specific work. General work would include lighter, more flowing strokes before working specifically with the deeper and more therapeutic techniques. Once the area has been prepared, the practitioner can then address any congestion, spasm, or ischemic conditions in the tissue that may be present. After the deeper and more specific work, the practitioner would return to general work in the area to normalize the tissue and help it recover.

IMPORTANCE OF DEVELOPING A SEQUENCE OF MASSAGE STROKES

Creating a sequence of massage strokes is important to both the practitioner's confidence and the client's comfort. A sequence gives the practitioner a structure from which to work and can be altered to allow for flexibility and creativity. The sequence also allows the massage to proceed in a logical fashion, which will provide comfort and relaxation to the client. This also ensures that every part of the body is massaged and each area is thoroughly covered. A sequence for a body part should start with gentle, light strokes to prepare the tissue; followed by deeper, more specific strokes that address problem areas within the tissue and decrease restrictions and increase range of motion. The deeper, more specific work should then be followed by lighter, more general strokes until the area is complete. The practitioner should also have a specific sequence in which the parts of the body are massaged in order to move around the body efficiently and logically, allowing the client to relax and feel comfortable.

MAINTAINING CONTACT WITH CLIENT AT ALL TIMES AND USING CONNECTING STROKES

The massage begins as soon as the practitioner lays his or her hands on a client's body. From that point, there must be constant contact with the client to ensure a continuous flow and assist the client in becoming relaxed and comfortable. If the client is alert with eyes open and is engaging in conversation with the practitioner, there is visual and verbal contact. If the client is in a state of relaxation and the eyes are closed, then visual contact cannot be maintained and verbal contact should only be made when necessary. It is important for the practitioner to maintain physical contact with the client so that there is an awareness of where the practitioner is and what to expect next. When the practitioner removes the hands then returns them to the body, it is stimulating to the client and disrupts relaxation. It can also make the massage feel inconsistent and without flow. If contact with the client must be broken, the practitioner should quietly inform the client, then remove the hands slowly and return them to the body gently so as not to surprise the client and remove them from the relaxed state.

EFFLEURAGE

Effleurage is a series of strokes that are applied through a gliding motion over an extended part of the body. It is the most frequently used stroke in Swedish massage. It comes from a French word meaning "to flow." It can be deep or superficial depending on the situation and intent of the massage. It can be performed with the palmar surface of the hand over larger areas or with the fingers in smaller areas. The gliding strokes of effleurage are used to spread lubricant on an area

Copyright © Mometrix Media. You have been licensed one copy of this document for personal use only. Any other reproduction or redistribution is strictly prohibited. All rights reserved. This content is provided for test preparation purposes only and does not imply an endorsement by Mometrix of any particular political, scientific, or religious point of view.

when beginning massage, as well as to prepare the tissue for deeper work. Effleurage will warm the tissue and enhance the blood and lymph flow. When done slowly, it has a calming effect; when done briskly, there is a stimulating effect. After deeper, more specific work is complete, effleurage can be used to remove waste from ischemic tissues by increasing circulation. Depending on the intent of the massage, the practitioner can then use effleurage to both soothe and calm the client before finishing the body part, or a brisker stroke can be applied to stimulate the area before moving on to the next body part.

GENERAL MASSAGE SEQUENCE

General massage sequence for any body part:

1. Undrape the body part and make contact
2. Use light effleurage to apply the lubricant
3. Use effleurage to allow the body to adjust to touch and flush the lymph and venous blood
4. Use kneading techniques such as petrissage to warm the tissues and feel for restricted areas
5. Use effleurage to flush the area
6. Use a friction technique to treat specific areas
7. Use deep gliding to areas in need of extra attention
8. Flush the entire area again with effleurage
9. Use joint movements to restore mobility and stretch the muscles and connective tissues and lubricate the joints
10. Use effleurage to flush the area and remove debris and give a feeling of length
11. Apply feathering strokes to end the work in that area and stimulate the nervous system
12. Re-drape the body part and continue to the next part

Hot/Cold Applications

CONTRAINDICATIONS FOR APPLYING HEAT AND COLD

Treatments involving either heat or cold should not be given to any client who is suffering cardiac impairment, diabetes, lung disease, kidney infection, extremely high or low blood pressure, any infectious skin condition, or open wound. If there is any impairment that could prevent the client from properly feeling hot or cold, then any treatments that could potentially burn or freeze the client's skin should be avoided. Warm or cool treatments would be considered safe. During pregnancy, a woman should not receive treatments that would raise the body's core temperature. Those with multiple sclerosis will have an increase in symptoms when the body temperature is elevated, so applications of heat should be avoided. If the client has any aversion to heat or cold, then the treatment should be avoided or discontinued. If there are any conditions that are considered questionable for hot or cold treatment, then the client's physician should be consulted. It is always best to use extreme caution when using applications of heat or cold on all clients, due to the risk of burning or freezing the skin or a client having a negative reaction.

PHYSIOLOGICAL EFFECTS OF COLD APPLICATIONS

Cold affects the body in two ways. First is an immediate and temporary effect followed by a secondary and more long-lasting effect. Cold will stimulate circulation, sedate the nerves, and slow the cells' metabolic activity. Prolonged use of cold will have a depressive effect, so caution is recommended. When cold is applied to the body, the immediate effects are a chilling of the skin; constriction of surface blood vessels, which drives blood to the interior of the body; a reduction in nerve sensitivity; a slowing of metabolic activity; and a reduction in inflammation and swelling. After the application of cold is removed, there is a secondary effect which is longer lasting. The skin will begin to warm and become relaxed and the surface blood vessels will dilate, which will bring

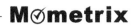

more blood to the skin. Nerve sensitivity will begin to increase and the surrounding cells will become more functionally active.

PHYSIOLOGICAL EFFECTS OF HEAT APPLICATIONS

Heat's effect on the body depends on the temperature, the duration of the treatment, and the area of the body being contacted by the heat source. The immediate effect of heat is the dilation of local blood vessels and capillaries, which will increase oxygen absorption and circulation and bring blood from the interior of the body to the surface. With long and continued application of heat, all skin functions will increase and there will be profuse sweating. Over time, pain and stiffness will be reduced and range of motion will increase. Heat will cause the superficial fascia to become softer and the collagen in the connective tissues will develop increased extensibility. Heat applications that are moderately warm will relax the muscles, blood vessels, and nerves, and increase the metabolic activity of the cells. Moist heat will tend to penetrate deeper into the muscles than dry heat, creating an increased relaxation effect to muscle tissue.

CONTRAST THERAPY

Contrast therapy is the application of alternating heat and cold. It is considered a very effective method of increasing local circulation by causing an alternating vasodilation and vasoconstriction of the blood vessels in the area. Increasing the circulation will relieve pain and stiffness from trauma and will stimulate the healing of injuries or wounds. A contrast bath will require two tubs. One tub will be filled with hot water of 104 degrees Fahrenheit. The other tub will be filled with cold or ice water. The body part should first be immersed in the hot water until the water no longer feels hot. When the body part adapts to the heat it is removed and placed in the cold water for 30 seconds to 2 minutes or until the client becomes accustomed to the cold. Hot water can be added to the hot bath while the client is completing the cold therapy in order to bring the water back up to temperature. The procedure is repeated three to six times, always finishing with cold.

ACCEPTABLE RANGE OF TEMPERATURES FOR USE IN HOT OR COLD THERAPY TREATMENTS

Normal body temperature is 98.6 degrees Fahrenheit. This is the temperature the body will attempt to maintain. Treatments that are applied to the body using heat or cold will cause certain physiological effects. Any treatment that is the same temperature as the body will have no thermal effects. Temperatures that are extreme should be avoided to prevent freezing or burning of the skin. Any treatments below freezing or above 115 degrees Fahrenheit can cause tissue damage. Treatments below 70 degrees Fahrenheit that are prolonged and general can cause hypothermia. Hyperthermia can be caused by prolonged general treatments at temperatures greater than 104 degrees Fahrenheit. Both of these conditions are dangerous. Temperatures for hydrotherapy applications of cold and heat should range from 56 degrees Fahrenheit, which can be uncomfortable and should not be used for long periods, to a maximum of 110 degrees Fahrenheit. Temperatures between 105-110 degrees Fahrenheit are tolerable for only short periods of time. Anything below 56 degrees Fahrenheit would be considered painful and should not be used unless under medical supervision.

Overview of Massage/Bodywork Modalities

SWEDISH MASSAGE

Swedish massage is based on the physiological insights of Per Henrik Ling. Presently, it is the most common form of massage practiced in the United States. It involves the use of the hands, elbows, and lower arms. During a Swedish massage, the flesh of the client is kneaded and vigorously manipulated in order to increase circulation, promote relaxation, and diminish stress. Swedish massage includes several different kinds of strokes: effleurage (long, superficial strokes); pétrissage (kneading); tapotement (gentle beating); and rubbing. Research consistently shows that Swedish massage increases the flow of blood and lymphatic fluid throughout the body.

NEUROMUSCULAR MASSAGE

Neuromuscular massage emphasizes pressure applied to the so-called "trigger points" on the body. Trigger points are areas where the nervous system can be stimulated through light touch. These points correspond to other areas of the body, which can be healed through attention to the trigger points. Neuromuscular massage typically entails applying moderate pressure to the trigger points for prolonged periods of time. The goals of neuromuscular therapy are to reduce pain, correct problems with posture, and enhance range of motion. The term "neuromuscular" reflects the attention this technique gives to the interrelationship between the nervous and muscular systems.

CIRCULATORY MASSAGE

Although most massage ends up improving the body's circulation, there are some modalities which have this as their central aim. The goal of circulatory massage is to improve the circulation of blood, lymphatic fluid, and waste products. Circulatory massage incorporates a variety of mechanical techniques that stimulate the flow of blood by improving the performance of arteries and veins. Also, there are a number of lymph drainage techniques that initiate the movement of lymph from the body tissues to the heart. A trained massage therapist will also be able to stimulate the evacuation of waste by applying specific types of pressure to the lower intestine.

ENERGY MASSAGE

Two of the most common forms of energy massage are Reiki and polarity therapy. Reiki aims to support the flow of energy throughout the body. The practice of Reiki is relatively easy to learn; very little formal training is required. Polarity therapy, meanwhile, seeks to improve health by making adjustments to the energy field that surrounds every human being. According to practitioners of polarity therapy, the natural circulation of electrical energy around the human body can be obstructed by imperfect body processes. These obstructions may be caused by poor posture, mood disorders, or muscular tension. The practitioner of polarity therapy tries to restore the electrical field around the subject so that he or she can regain normal energy flow.

MOVEMENT MASSAGE

Movement massage modalities oblige the client to take a more active role in his or her therapy. Some of the most common varieties of movement massage are Feldenkrais, Trager, and Alexander. Feldenkrais emphasizes relearning common movement patterns in such a way that they diminish the stresses placed on certain parts of the body. The Alexander technique is specifically aimed at improving posture and balance by forcing the client to become conscious of habitual movements. This method is especially popular among actors and dancers because of the control it gives the client over his or her body. The Trager system encourages clients to move their bodies as a therapist applies light pressure to certain key areas; this technique is good for relieving muscular tension.

STRUCTURAL AND POSTURAL INTEGRATION MASSAGE AND BODYWORK

Structural and postural integration modalities emphasize the importance of developing and maintaining proper body alignment when standing and performing normal movements. Two of the most common modalities in this category are Rolfing and Hellerwork. Rolfing focuses on improving posture through a systematic reshaping of the body's myofascial structure. A certified "Rolfer" administers light pressure all over the body with his or her fingers, elbows, and knuckles. The goal is to relax the muscles until they reach their natural state of alignment. Hellerwork, meanwhile,

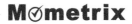

focuses on releasing built-up tension in the connective tissues. According to this discipline, the body becomes used to destructive misalignment, and requires massage to regain its natural structure.

ORIENTAL MASSAGE

Oriental massage modalities emphasize the flow of energy through the body. According to their theories, the unrestricted flow of energy supports good health. Some of the most common modalities in this category are Acupressure and Shiatsu massage. Acupressure, as the name indicates, is a combination of acupuncture and massage. It involves the application of light pressure to the points of the body which, in acupuncture, are pierced with needles. Shiatsu is a similar therapy that involves treating the entire body. Shiatsu theory asserts that by restoring the overall health of the body, particular areas of stress and tension can be alleviated. Shiatsu involves the application of light pressure to the acupuncture sites in the hope that it will restore effective energy flow through the body.

REFLEXOLOGY

Reflexology is a study that involves stimulating certain parts of the body to produce a reaction in other parts of the body. It is based on the principal that every organ within the body has a corresponding point on either the hands or feet. By applying pressure to the ball of the foot, for example, the practitioner can produce a favorable reaction within the lungs and heart. In addition to the organs, reflexology can also affect glands and muscles. Through the application of pressure to the areas corresponding to these glands, tension can be relieved, and there may be an overall increase in body function. As an example, the heel of the foot is believed to correspond to the lower back. Pressure on the big toe can lead to relief from headaches. It is important to understand that some skeptics do not believe that this type of massage is beneficial. In any case, practitioners should not project the opinion that reflexology is a medical cure-all.

CHAIR MASSAGE

Chair massage originated in Japan, and is believed to be several centuries old. It is a form of massage that has become increasingly popular. It can be found in shopping malls, airports, workplaces, convention centers, and other areas where large numbers of people congregate. Chair massage allows the client to be fully clothed while sitting in a chair in a semi-reclined, prone position. Chair massage is an effective way to introduce massage to a person who may exhibit adverse reactions to touch, and is also suitable for those who may consider traditional Swedish massage too invasive.

ADVANTAGES

Chair massage is often an introduction to massage therapy for individuals who, for one reason or another, are apprehensive about the process. Chair massage is sometimes used as a way to introduce positive reactions to touch. It may be suitable for those who have been victims of sexual, physical, or emotional abuse. The chair massage technique enables the practitioner to complete a session in less than 30 minutes, thus making it readily accessible to those on a tight schedule. Finally, chair massage is more cost-effective than standard massage sessions, allowing it to be used by people who are less inclined or able to spend money on weekly massages.

PROCEDURE

Due to the high volume of massages being performed by chair massage practitioners, the initial consultation will likely be shorter than in a standard therapeutic setting. However, the practitioner should still screen for any contraindications to the massage prior to commencement. As the client is fully clothed and seated in a prone position, certain techniques, including effleurage and gliding, are not possible. Due to the nature of chair massage, friction, percussion, and deep touches are the only

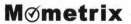

appropriate techniques. With the client seated in the prone position, the head, neck, shoulders, back, and hips may be the only areas the practitioner can access.

SPECIAL CONSIDERATIONS AND HYGIENIC PRACTICES

Some chair massages require the therapist to take special considerations into account in order to provide adequate therapeutic benefits to the client. In some cases, the client is seated in a supine position to enable the therapist to gain access to the lower legs and feet to perform massage in those areas. After each client leaves, the practitioner must ensure the chair meets standards of cleanliness before the next client is seated. Wiping down areas that come into contact with the client's skin with an anti-bacterial cleanser is important to control transmission of bacteria or germs. As an alternative, disposable coverings for the face cushion can be used.

LYMPH MASSAGE

Lymph massage is closely related to Swedish massage. It is designed to assist with the movement of the lymphatic fluids within the body. When lymph nodes are filled with fluid, a condition known as lymphedema, physicians sometimes recommend lymph drainage massage as a means of alleviating the symptoms. Specific methods designed to assist with the flow of lymph fluids can cause an increase in metabolism, drain stagnant fluids and toxins, and stimulate the immune system. The rhythmic movements used in lymph massage also stimulate the parasympathetic nervous system which, in turn, helps to relieve stress, depression, and insomnia. Lymph massage can also help rebalance the chemistry within the body, assist in tissue regeneration, normalize organs, and boost the immune system. When done correctly, the procedure entails gentle, slow movements that are performed over the lymph nodes in a circular pattern. Light pressure is then applied in the direction of lymph flow to direct the movement of lymph.

DEEP TISSUE MASSAGE

Deep tissue massage targets the tissues of the body that are below the superficial musculature. Some of the most common forms of deep tissue massage include cross-fiber friction, connective tissue massage, craniosacral massage, and myofascial massage. A deep tissue massage generally includes long strokes of moderate intensity and prolonged periods of pressure to certain points on the body. In order to apply direct contact to the deep muscles of the body, a certain degree of relaxation must be achieved. Therefore, it may take a while before attention can be directed to the deep muscles. Deep tissue massage can be painful, so the client should be monitored closely during each session. Deep tissue massage refers to the massage style that focuses on the deeper muscles and fascia tissues. Various techniques are used in this form of massage to alleviate any tension in the muscular fibers. Massage of this nature can also contribute to psychological and physiological changes in the body. These therapeutic techniques may require long warm-up periods before the deep tissues of the client can be accessed. The intent behind this type of massage is to loosen the bonds between the layers of connective tissue. Some of the popular deep massage techniques are Rolfing, Trager, Hellerwork, and Feldenkrais.

ROLFING

One type of deep tissue massage, known as Rolfing, is named after Dr. Ida Rolf, the woman who developed the technique. She devised this technique to alleviate tension and structural problems caused by years of poor posture and alignment. Rolfing utilizes a heavy-handed technique to realign the body. Performed over a series of many treatments, the massage therapist uses his or her hands, fists, or even knuckles to align the body's movements and create a sense of balance within. A full treatment of Rolfing involves a series of 10 treatments, although fewer treatments can also lead to improvement.

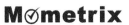

TRIGGER POINT THERAPY

Trigger points in the body refer to skeletal muscle areas that are hyperirritable. The presence of palpable nodules in the bands of muscle fibers sometimes causes pain responses that can refer to other parts of the body. Trigger points are classified according to their location in the body and whether or not pain is felt upon palpitation. A common trigger point site is an acupuncture site, though some trigger points are located elsewhere on the body. Activation of a trigger point can be caused by an increase in stress levels, overuse of a particular muscle, and even an arthritic condition. A brief listing of common trigger points is given below:

- Active myofascial trigger point
- Latent myofascial trigger point
- Central trigger point
- Attachment trigger point
- Primary (or key) trigger point
- Satellite trigger point
- Associate trigger point

ACUPRESSURE

Similar in theory to acupuncture, acupressure is a Chinese technique in which pressure is applied from the hand, elbow, or fingers to acupuncture points across the body. The purpose of acupressure is to relieve the body by balancing the physical and psychological aspects. Through this method, a person can experience an increase in circulatory function and an enhanced ability to manage pain. Acupressure is usually part of an overall health regimen that also incorporates a healthy diet, exercise, and meditation. The overall goal is to develop a holistic lifestyle. Areas of the body where pressure points may be found are along the crown of the head, the temple, the forehead, and the upper jaw. Other areas can include the sides and front of the neck, upper arms, elbow joint, and the outside of the thighs and lower legs. Areas that commonly experience feelings of relief through acupressure include the toes, metatarsals, ankles, heels, and Achilles tendon.

HYDROTHERAPY

Hydrotherapy is the practice of using water in its liquid, gas, or solid forms as part of a massage therapy treatment plan. Heat therapy can involve the application of dry heat, moist heat, or diathermy. Dry heat involves the use of heating pads, infrared radiation, or a sauna. Moist heat can come from an immersion bath, spray, heat packs, or a steam bath. Diathermy can entail the transmission of shortwave or microwave electromagnetic fields onto the tissue. The purpose of heat therapy is to cause vessels to dilate and increase circulation. Care must be taken to closely monitor the client's body temperature. Cold therapy is also known as cryotherapy. This technique is performed to help reduce the edema, swelling, and pain accompanying an injury. Cold treatments should be applied for short periods of time due to the possibility of tissue injury from the cold. Examples of cold treatments are immersion baths, ice packs, ice massage, mechanical compressors, and vasocoolant sprays.

When used as a method of therapy, water can be used in any of its three forms: solid, liquid, or gaseous vapor. When cold water is used for hydrotherapy, it has the immediate effect of cooling the skin and drawing blood away from the surface of the body. The nerves experience a reduction in their sensitivity levels and the activity of the body's cells in that particular area begins to slow down. After these initial reactions take place, a secondary reaction occurs, which causes the skin to become warmer and more relaxed. The blood cells on the surface of the skin begin to expand again; nerve impulses increase. The activity level of nearby cells increases. When heat therapy is conducted, reactions that occur cause the blood cells from the interior of the body to move towards

111

the surface of the skin, which produces a reddish area on the skin. These blood vessels dilate and cause an increase in circulation. The body's temperature rises, and sweating may occur. All of these changes serve to relax the blood vessels, nerves, and muscles.

AROMATHERAPY

Aromatherapy is the use of essential oils from natural herbs, flowers, and spices to enhance the massage experience through the sense of smell. These aromas can bring about a specific reaction, and are commonly chosen to augment the massage session. Some of the most popular essential oils are chamomile, eucalyptus, jasmine, lavender, and lemongrass. The effects these oils produce can be calming, stimulating, refreshing, or relaxing. It is not a good idea to use these essential oils at their full strength. Instead, they should be combined with another medium, such as carrier oil. This oil serves as a lubricant, and helps to blend the oil so it is not overly concentrated, which can cause irritation. Aromatherapy can also involve the use of scented candles or lotion. Prior to the massage, the therapist should consult the intake form or ask the client verbally about any allergies or sensitivities to oils or aromas that may be used during the massage.

BODY WRAPS

Body wraps are used for different purposes, including relaxation, detoxification, and cleansing and softening the skin. Various substances can be used in the wraps, including seaweed, volcanic clay, and mud. Heat is a common element of wraps, whether it comes from an outside source or is obtained from the body. Contraindicators for wraps include high blood pressure, heart disease, and pregnancy. Body wraps are beneficial in that they provide comfort, security, and warmth, and also allow the nutrients to be absorbed in a closed environment instead of being dispersed through the air.

TECHNIQUE

When performing a body wrap, the practitioner must be aware of factors that may prevent the client from being fully wrapped. The practitioner must also take precautions when determining the temperature level of the wrap. The table is laid out with a blanket, a thermal blanket, a towel, and finally, a plastic wrap. The client lies down on this plastic, and an exfoliation is performed on the client's skin prior to the application of the seaweed or mud. As the seaweed or mud is brushed over the body, the practitioner wraps that portion of the body to prevent heat from escaping. Upon completion, the client is completely engulfed in wraps, and is allowed to relax for some time before being assisted through the clean-up process by the therapist.

EXFOLIATION PROCEDURE

An exfoliation procedure can be performed in a massage therapy room. In this instance, the body is moistened with a sponge rather than in a shower or bath. After the body has been moistened, the practitioner puts salts or exfoliates into his hands and applies them in a circular fashion over the body. Only one surface is exfoliated at a time. A wet towel is used to wipe off the salts, and then a wet loofah is used to apply soap to the body. After the body has been cleansed, another hot, wet cloth is used to remove all residue of soap. The body is then dried off with another towel, and the practitioner then applies moisturizer all over the body. Exfoliation using salts from the Dead Sea is similar in nature, except the salts are mixed with water to form a paste prior to applying them to the body.

ATHLETIC OR SPORTS MASSAGE

Athletic massage is used to help treat athletic injuries, which increases the level of strength training, conditioning, and activity. The sports massage therapist must be knowledgeable about anatomy, physiology, kinesiology, and biomechanics in order to help the athlete return to the level

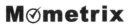

of conditioning required for his sport. Biomechanics refers to the movement of the body. Soft tissue injuries commonly account for a large portion of the injuries seen by the sports massage therapist. Sports massage therapists must have knowledge of the various muscle groups and how they are used within the sport. It is also important for him to understand the functions of the circulatory system and the nervous system, as they also interact with the muscles.

BENEFICIAL EFFECTS

The main effects of an athletic massage are:

- Oxygen is more readily available, which allows for repair of the injured body part.
- Waste materials are flushed out by increased circulation, causing increased energy levels.
- The muscles, ligaments, and tendons are stretched, allowing for greater flexibility.
- The occurrence of muscle spasms is reduced.
- Adhesions are broken down within the muscle, resulting in less scar tissue formation after an injury.
- Collagen fibers come into alignment, leading to a stronger healed area.
- The likelihood of future injuries is reduced.
- Acids are released from the body, which causes the muscles to "bounce" back after an intense workout.
- The career of an athlete can potentially be extended because they may sustain fewer injuries.

BENEFITS IN A REHABILITATION SITUATION

When performing a warm-up massage on an athlete, it is important to note any potential problems that could lead to a more serious, debilitating injury. If an injury does occur, massage can help to alleviate the common problems associated with the injury. Massage is an effective means of reducing edema and swelling of the affected joint or area. The time that the body needs to recover from the injury is minimized. The scar tissue that is formed at the site of the injury is more flexible, which means the tissue is less stiff. The athlete can develop an increased range of motion in the affected limb as a result of continued massage. The athlete stands a greater chance of returning to full form more quickly than if massage was not included as part of the rehabilitation program.

COMPONENTS

An athletic massage is broken down into four parts: pre-event massage, post-event massage, restorative or training massage, and rehabilitation massage. Pre-event massage is used before a competition to prepare and invigorate the athlete for the rigors of a competition. It is usually given between 15 minutes to 4 hours before a competition to increase flexibility and circulation. A post-event massage helps to cool the body down and restore the tissues to their normal state. The kneading, compression, and light stretching also helps to relax the athlete. A restorative massage is used during training, and includes deep cross-fiber friction and joint stretches. Rehabilitation massage is used to help heal and repair muscle tissue after an injury. This type of massage shortens the recuperative time and also prevents any scar tissue from forming. It helps build a stronger muscle or joint, and also allows the athlete to return to training with less likelihood of re-injury.

Client Assessment, Reassessment, and Treatment Planning

Organization of a Massage/Bodywork Session

PREPARING A SPACE TO DO MASSAGE

The most important considerations that go into choosing a massage space are insuring the comfort and safety of both the client and practitioner. There must be easy access into and out of the space so that a client who is elderly or has special needs will have no difficulties accessing the massage table. There should also be a location for the client to leave personal belongings and a chair to sit in to remove shoes and clothes. In order for the practitioner to be comfortable, the space should have adequate room to move around the table and storage for supplies that have easy access for anything that could be needed during the massage. Lighting should be bright enough to allow both client and practitioner to see the space, but also soft and soothing to maintain the massage environment. Controls to adjust the room temperature are also vital to maintaining client comfort during the massage session.

PRODUCTS AND SUPPLIES NECESSARY FOR MASSAGE

List of supplies needed in the massage room:

- Massage table
- Stool for therapist
- Tissues for client's convenience
- Clock
- Bolsters
- Cleaning and sanitizing products
- Wastebasket
- Face cradle covers
- Linens and blankets
- Chair or stool for the client
- Lubricants and oils or creams
- Music player
- Pillows
- Towels
- Bolster covers
- Lighting
- A mirror so clients can check appearance before leaving room
- Personal hygiene products so clients can freshen up

Client Consultation and Evaluation

DETERMINING NEEDS AND EXPECTATIONS OF CLIENTS

The consultation, which is the initial interview, is the best time to assess and determine what the client needs and expects from the massage session. In order to make the consultation as productive as possible, it is important for the practitioner to listen carefully to the client and develop an interview style that adapts to the client's level of intelligence and knowledge of massage. Some

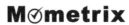

clients may need to see the information in writing and have the practitioner go over the material, while others will best understand the information through a verbal explanation. It is important to maintain eye contact and use the client's name during the conversation in order to develop a rapport. When a client feels comfortable, it is more likely that the conversation will be open and productive. Mimicking the client's body language will also help the client to feel accepted and confident during the consultation. The most important aspect, however, is listening intently to what the client is reporting and responding accordingly.

PREPARING A CLIENT FOR A MASSAGE SESSION

The first step in preparing a client for a massage session would be to have the client complete all necessary paperwork, then follow that with a comprehensive consultation of which the goal would be to understand the client's needs and expectations for the massage session. It is important to inform the client of all policies and procedures and to thoroughly check over and discuss the intake form. The practitioner should then perform a preliminary assessment and document any postural abnormalities or areas of concern. During this time, the practitioner should be carefully assessing for any contraindications. Once it is determined that the client may receive massage and that all policies and procedures are understood, the practitioner may then show the client to the massage room and explain the process of disrobing and getting on to the massage table as well as what will happen during the massage so the client has a full understanding of the entire process.

ASSISTING CLIENTS ON/OFF OF THE MASSAGE TABLE

If a client presents with a disability, is frail and/or elderly, or of very small stature, then it would be appropriate for the practitioner to offer assistance both on to and off of the massage table. Because many clients choose to disrobe, the offer of assistance may be turned down due to modesty concerns. The practitioner may have a robe available for clients to change into before receiving assistance on to the table or may choose to perform the massage session through the clothes if the client is unable to undress and get on to the massage table unassisted. If a client shows any signs of experiencing lightheadedness or dizziness after the session, or if the client has a history of low blood pressure or problems with balance, then it is recommended that the practitioner offer assistance in getting up from the table and returning to a standing position. It is also recommended that a practitioner have a stool available so that clients who are of small stature or elderly can use it to step up as they climb on to the table.

PROPER DRAPING TECHNIQUE

Proper draping will allow the client to remain covered, warm, and feel safe and comfortable during the massage.

- **Top Cover Method** – This method uses two coverings, one to cover the table and one to cover the entire body. During the massage, only the body part that is being massaged should be exposed and the portion of the sheet not covering the body should be tucked under the part being massaged. When rolling the client over, the practitioner should secure the sheet by leaning the hips into the table and grasping the top sheet at the level of the client's shoulders and hips, then holding the sheet up just enough for the client to roll over. The client should always roll towards the practitioner to avoid rolling off of the table.

Client Assessment, Reassessment, and Treatment Planning

115

Copyright © Mometrix Media. You have been licensed one copy of this document for personal use only. Any other reproduction or redistribution is strictly prohibited. All rights reserved. This content is provided for test preparation purposes only and does not imply an endorsement by Mometrix of any particular political, scientific, or religious point of view.

- **Full Sheet Draping** – One double-size flat sheet is used to cover both table and client. The client wears a wrap from the dressing area to the table. Once the client is on the table, the practitioner will fold one side of the sheet over the client's entire torso and one leg. At this time, the wrap can be removed. The other half of the sheet is then draped over the entire torso and the opposite leg. During massage of the legs, it is only necessary to pull back one section of sheet. The portion draping the opposite leg can then be tucked under the thigh of the leg being massaged in order to ensure modesty. In order for the client to roll over, the wrap can be used to cover the body. Be sure to have the client roll toward the practitioner for safety. Draping for massage of the back of the legs would be the same as the front. To massage the back, the practitioner would carefully peel down the draping without exposing the gluteal area.

CLIENT CONSULTATIONS

NONVERBAL COMMUNICATION IN THE CLIENT CONSULTATION

Nonverbal communication is body language. It includes posture, facial expressions, gestures, and other nonverbal clues as to what a person may be thinking or feeling. Oftentimes, the clues picked up from body language can be more informative than the verbal conversation. During the consultation, if the practitioner notices that the client's body language does not coincide with what is being verbally communicated, then this would be a sign that the client may feel uncomfortable or may not be telling how they truly feel. Sometimes clients will say that they are feeling fine, but their body language may tell a different story. It is important for the practitioner to be perceptive and pay attention to both nonverbal and verbal clues. Sensing that the client may not be disclosing the full information could lead the practitioner to change the format of the questioning, which may allow the client to be more forthcoming. The practitioner's nonverbal communication is also important to the comfort of the client. Leaning forward, smiling, and allowing the body to remain at ease are all ways to communicate confidence and comfort to the client, which in turn will allow the client to relax and be more open.

INFORMATION TO GATHER DURING CONSULTATION

The practitioner's goals during the consultation are to learn as much as possible about the client's needs and expectations for the massage, any pertinent conditions or concerns, and what types of treatments they may have received before. The practitioner should ask open-ended questions so as to allow the client to expand on their answers and provide as much information as possible. The practitioner is attempting to learn what the client foresees as the result of the session and gathering information that will assist in creating a treatment plan. Setting goals for what the client expects to achieve should also be a part of the consultation. Any possible contraindications should also be addressed during the consultation and the practitioner should take this time to explain the procedures for the massage. There should be an exchange of information that will allow the practitioner to provide the best service possible and for the client to feel comfortable and have enough information to provide informed consent for the massage.

DEVELOPMENT OF TREATMENT PLAN

A treatment plan gives the practitioner an outline for providing treatment. It can cover one individual session or a longer-term series of treatments. The treatment plan is developed based on the information provided in the consultation and from the intake and health history forms. The practitioner will review all of the information provided by the client as well as information obtained during the interview and initial assessment. This information will allow the practitioner to ascertain if there are any contraindications which would require a referral to a physician or any changes to the treatment plan. The practitioner is also looking for indications of which techniques and modalities would be most effective for achieving the goals and results that were agreed upon in

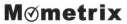

the consultation. The treatment plan should be reviewed and revised based on the results of each individual session and feedback from the client. The treatment plan should be developed and explained to the client beforehand so that informed consent can be given regarding the plan for treatment and how it will be put in to action.

HEALTH HISTORY FORM

The primary importance of the health history form is to give the practitioner information on the client's past and present health issues so that the practitioner is able to devise an appropriate treatment plan and have a full understanding of the client's health. The health history form will also inquire about any possible contraindications so that the practitioner can request further information and make an informed decision about whether massage is indicated and whether a referral is required. The health history form will save the practitioner time during the initial consultation. The health history form should be signed by the client stating it is accurate. This could protect the practitioner from liability issues if it is discovered that the client did not divulge a health issue that could be a contraindication for massage. The form will also allow the practitioner to review client information before future sessions. It is important for the practitioner to interview the client and request elaboration on any answers that may require further consideration.

INFORMATION INCLUDED

The health history form gives the massage practitioner a very important overview of a client's health history. This form should first include demographic information such as age, weight, height, and emergency contact information. The form should then provide a thorough history of any conditions that would be pertinent to the massage practitioner. Information on the client's history of massage would be important to gather. The practitioner should know if the client has had a massage before and how often. There should be space for the client to enter current complaints and the reasons for seeking a massage. Provide the client with a comprehensive list of diseases and conditions that could be contraindications or may affect the massage. It is also important to include a lifestyle section asking the client about such things as type of employment, sports or activities involved in, stress level, and any hobbies or activities that may involve repetitive stress. The practitioner should also include questions regarding skin sensitivities and allergies so that appropriate massage lubricant is used during a session.

UNFAMILIAR ILLNESS

If a client presents with an illness that is unfamiliar, the practitioner should attempt to become educated on this condition. The first thing the practitioner should do is ask the client to explain the condition and inquire whether massage has been received in the past. Many times, the client will be able to educate the practitioner about the condition and if massage would be appropriate. Depending on the type of condition, the practitioner would have to make an informed decision about whether massage is indicated. The practitioner could use a resource to research the condition and receive more in-depth information. Should there not be enough information available, or if the client has never received massage before, then it is recommended that the client return at a later date with a letter from their treating physician stating that massage is indicated. It is important for the practitioner to set a strict boundary in this type of case because the client is often motivated to receive the massage immediately and may refuse to provide a doctor's referral. It is most important to do no harm and not provide a massage treatment that would be contraindicated.

117

Written Data Collection

ACCURATE CLIENT RECORDS

Client records are an important way for the practitioner to document the work that has been done with a client and the results that have been achieved. If a practitioner does not keep accurate records, it will be difficult to measure the effectiveness of the results. By referring back to the initial consultation and assessment, the practitioner will have a measurable record of improvement gains. Sometimes, clients do not return for massage for long periods of time, so having an accurate record to reflect back on can assist the practitioner in recalling the previous treatments with the client and can also serve to demonstrate what may or may not have been effective in the past. Maintaining proper records can also protect a practitioner in the event of litigation and is an important basis of communication when dealing with other health care professionals. Keeping accurate and complete records can be tedious, but it is an essential part of running a professional massage practice.

SOAP CHARTING

SOAP charting is the most popular way for a practitioner to format the recording of client session information. SOAP stands for "subjective, objective, assessment or application, and planning." SOAP charts should be used to document information from the initial interview and assessment, as well as each individual treatment session.

- **Subjective** – This section contains information that the client has reported. This could include pain levels, health history, present condition, how the condition started, any aggravating factors, as well as anything that improves the condition. This information should be updated at each session.
- **Objective** – This section contains the observations of the therapist. Objective descriptions are generally more measurable. For example, range of motion is objective. The practitioner should record results from the assessment in this section.
- **Assessment** or **Application** – This section is where notes about what treatment was used in the session and any changes that might have occurred due to the treatment are recorded. The practitioner should record all outcomes and relate those to the session goals.
- **Planning** – The planning section gives the practitioner a place to record notes regarding future sessions and long-range goals. The practitioner should also record any suggestions or recommendations for follow-up that were given to the client.

The **S** in SOAP chart stands for "**subjective**." This portion of the SOAP chart is where the massage practitioner documents the findings from the initial interview and intake. This includes anything that the client reports to the practitioner, such as health history, current symptoms, aggravating conditions, any activities or therapies that have made the condition better or worse, and how the condition started. This information can come from the interview and the intake forms, as well as anything that may be reported during the massage. This information should be updated at each session so that the present condition is reported. If using a pain scale to document the client's progress, it should be reported in this section. A client's goals and expectations for the massage treatments should be documented in this section as well. If the practitioner is billing insurance for the massage sessions, it is important that the documentation of all subjective findings correspond to the diagnosis on the prescription provided by the medical practitioner.

The **O** in SOAP chart stands for "**objective**." This portion of the SOAP chart is where the massage practitioner documents the findings from the observation and interview with the client and any assessments or tests that have been done. These would be the practitioner's objective findings. Information from this section is used to outline the treatment goals. If the practitioner finds any

118

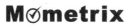

abnormalities in the client's gait or posture, or notices anything abnormal during the massage, this should be reported in the objective section. All range of motion tests, both active and passive, should be documented in this section as well. This section will often contain body diagrams where the practitioner can make notes or draw graphics to show postural abnormalities. If the practitioner is billing insurance for the massage sessions, then it is important that the documentation of all objective findings correspond to the diagnosis on the prescription provided by the medical practitioner.

MAINTAINING CLIENT CONFIDENTIALITY

In order to maintain client confidentiality, the practitioner must ensure that all client files are kept secure and should be visible only to those who need to see the file for treatment or billing purposes. If information needs to be shared with a third party, the practitioner should obtain written consent from the client. The written consent form giving permission to share client information should contain the practitioner's name, the client's name, and the name of the third party who will be receiving the information. The form should contain a time frame in which the information may be released. The form should be signed and dated and kept in the client file. If client files are kept electronically, the practitioner should have these files password protected and use appropriate firewalls to protect from Internet access risks. All files and appointment books with client names and contact information should be kept out of the view of others and not left in the open. It is recommended that the practitioner create a privacy policy for the practice and have each client read and sign the document.

Visual Assessment

VISUAL OBSERVATIONS TO MAKE WHEN CLIENT WALKS THROUGH THE DOOR

The practitioner should be observing the client as soon as they walk through the door. Observation of the client's body language can provide valuable information to the practitioner. Looking at how the client walks, moves, sits, and stands can provide insight into what might be causing any pain the client is feeling. Observing the client closely can also give the practitioner clues as to the client's emotional state and personality, which can prove helpful in interactions during the interview. The practitioner should also look for any issues related to balance and gait that could indicate disease or disorder. Comparing one side of the body with the other is helpful in locating areas of tension or dysfunction. Observing posture is extremely important because it can provide information about muscular imbalances or structural deviations. All of this can be ascertained by using the simple skill of observation during normal interactions with the client.

CONTINUING VISUAL ASSESSMENT WHILE PERFORMING THE MASSAGE

It is important to continue to visually assess a client while performing a massage because there will be visual clues as to how effective the massage is as well as how the client is responding to the treatment. A practitioner should be taking note of the client's body temperature, tissue condition, and body language during the entire massage. Subtle movements or facial expressions may indicate a client's discomfort or pleasure with the techniques being used. The practitioner should be looking to continuously solicit feedback for the duration of the massage. Changes in temperature, texture, and moisture on the skin can indicate whether a particular treatment plan is working or will need to be adjusted. A practitioner who stays in tune visually throughout the massage will be able to better serve the client by making adjustments and modifications as needed in order to provide the best possible treatment.

Client Assessment, Reassessment, and Treatment Planning

USING A PLUMB LINE AND WALL CHART GRID FOR POSTURAL ASSESSMENT

A plumb line and wall chart grid are used to measure a client's static posture. To use a plumb line, the practitioner hangs a rope or cord with a plumb bob (small lead weight) that sits about three inches above the floor. Specific bony landmarks can then be vertically assessed against the plumb line. When observing the client either anteriorly or posteriorly, the plumb bob should sit midway between the heels. When viewing the client laterally, the plumb bob should sit just anterior to the lateral malleolus. The practitioner can then visually observe for any indications of muscular imbalances. The wall chart grid can be used in conjunction with the plumb line. It is placed on the wall and the client stands in front of the grid. A wall grid is best used to observe the level of the hips and shoulders. Together, the plumb line and wall chart grid can give the practitioner an excellent tool for measuring postural discrepancies.

CAUSES OF POSTURAL DISTORTION

Common causes of postural distortion:

- **Physical or emotional trauma** – Someone who has been injured physically may alter posture in order to protect the injured area and prevent further injury. Emotional trauma can also cause someone to change their posture. Often a more protective type of posture will develop, which may include forward rolling of shoulders and a forward head position.
- **Poor work habits** – Having a job that requires repetitive movements can cause a person to develop poor posture. Sitting at a desk for long periods in a poor position can cause muscle and fascia to tighten and restrict proper posture.
- **Pathologic conditions** – Certain diseases and disorders can cause changes in posture.
- **Age** – As people age, their posture tends to become more out of balance due to muscle loss and lack of activity.
- **Muscular imbalances** – When opposing muscle groups are out of balance, the posture can be affected.

USING BONY LANDMARKS TO ASSESS POSTURAL SYMMETRY

The body should be assessed from all four sides with the client standing erect. Starting from the bottom, the practitioner should observe the symmetry of the ankles, fibular heads, greater trochanter, iliac crests, scapula, acromioclavicular joints, and ears. The practitioner should also observe the patellae, the Achilles tendons, and the pelvis. The Achilles tendons should be perpendicular to the floor, the patellae should point forward, and the pelvis should be free of rotation and even. Using a plumb line, the practitioner can check that the ear, shoulder, elbow, acetabulum, knee, and ankle are in alignment. One side should not be higher than the other when viewed anteriorly or posteriorly, and there should be no rotation. Check for the position of the ears over the shoulders to assess whether there is a forward head posture or distortion at the neck. Viewing the body anteriorly should find the pubic symphysis, manubrium, and front of the zygomatic arch vertically aligned.

Palpation Assessment

PALPATION

Palpation is the primary assessment tool used by massage practitioners. It is a way to listen to the body through the hands and is an art that takes time to develop. Palpation can allow the practitioner to sense even the slightest changes in temperature, texture, moisture, and density of the tissues being palpated. The difference between normal and abnormal tissue can be felt and the therapist should be able to identify bony structures, individual muscles and any tight bands within

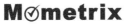

them, and skeletal alignment. Palpation should also identify areas of spasm, constriction, tight bands, or trigger points. Palpation can be done at any level from superficial to deep and through all types of tissue. The observations that a practitioner makes during palpation are both subjective and objective and should be used in conjunction with the consultation and range of motion testing to give a more complete picture of the client's condition.

INFORMATION LEARNED THROUGH PALPATION

There are a variety of different types of information that can be ascertained through palpation.

- **Temperature** – Tissue temperature that is outside the range of normal can be indicative of problems. Tissue that is cold may be having issues with vascular flow and tissue that is warm to the touch may indicate inflammation.
- **Texture** – The texture of tissue can vary quite a bit from one person to the next. Such things as cracking, splitting, dryness, sores, or rashes on the skin can indicate any number of disorders or conditions. Edema, scar tissue, fibrosis, cysts, or tumors may also be felt below the superficial level.
- **Tenderness** – Pain and tenderness felt in an area being palpated is a good sign that there is some type of dysfunction in the tissue.
- **Tone** – Hypertonic or hypotonic muscles can be felt through palpation and provide information on the state of the muscle tissue.
- **Referred sensation** – Myofascial trigger points or sensations from peripheral nerves can be activated during palpation.

IMPORTANCE OF APPROPRIATE PRESSURE

Palpation is a skill that is developed over time. Learning the appropriate pressure to use on varying structures and depths is an art that can be learned using basic guidelines. The biggest mistake that inexperienced practitioners make is using excessive pressure. At times, there is the need to use heavier pressure in order to access deeper tissue levels, but in most cases, palpation is more effective using lighter pressure. If there is a need to use deeper pressure, the practitioner should slowly and gently work the tissue from superficial toward deep until the desired tissue level is reached. Attempting to reach a deeper level too quickly can cause the client to stiffen and tighten the muscles and prevent further palpation. It is important to remember that palpation is used to observe and learn about the condition of the tissues, not to treat. Palpation should be strong enough to assess the desired tissues without affecting any kind of change in the tissue.

Client Assessment, Reassessment, and Treatment Planning

Range of Motion Assessment

END FEELS

End feel is the change in the feeling of the tissue at end of a joint movement.

Types of end feel:

- **Hard end feel** – This end feel occurs when there is bone-on-bone contact at the end of the range of motion. This is a normal end feel. An example would be full extension at the elbow joint.
- **Soft end feel** – The practitioner will start to feel a tightening and springiness of the tissues. This means the end of the range of motion is being reached. This is a cushioned end feel that is restricted from further movement by soft tissue. There should be no pain at this end feel.
- **Empty end feel** – When there is a sudden restriction to the range of motion before reaching the natural physiological barrier, this is known as an empty end feel. This end feel is usually due to pain and would be considered abnormal.

PHYSIOLOGICAL AND ANATOMIC BARRIERS

It is important for the practitioner to understand and recognize soft tissue barriers when assessing and treating clients. When a practitioner is moving a client's limb through a range of motion, there will be barriers to how far the movement can be completed. The physiological barrier is the barrier that is reached after the limb has been taken close to its full range of motion and the tissues have been stretched. At this point, the client may feel that the limb can go no further and some force is required to complete the stretch. If a practitioner would push further through this barrier, the anatomic barrier would be reached. The anatomic barrier is the point where the tissues have been maximally stretched and going past this point could cause tissue damage. Moving from the physiological barrier to the anatomic barrier could cause discomfort for the client. Depending on the health of the tissue, it is possible to move past the physiological barrier to the anatomic barrier with ease. If the client has any restrictions in the tissue, then the physiological barrier may be the maximum range of motion that can be reached without causing considerable discomfort.

Clinical Reasoning

RESPONSE TO CLIENT INJURY

A client arrives to a massage session and reports that on the previous day they fell on the ice and injured their shoulder. The client has been having considerable pain and has not yet consulted a physician. They are hoping that a massage will provide relief.

If a client arrives to a massage session with an injury that has not yet been seen by a physician, it is highly recommended that the practitioner defers the massage until the client has had the opportunity to be seen and treated by a physician, especially when the client is in considerable pain. If the client's only pain is in the shoulder and there are no other signs of injury, it would be up to the practitioner's discretion to consider all of the factors and choose whether to do a light massage that does not involve the shoulder. Factors to be considered would be the history with the client, other health conditions, relationship with the client, and extent of the injury based on assessment. It is always in the best interest of the client, despite their protests, to insist on the clearance of a physician if there is any doubt as to the extent of an injury.

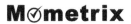

SETTING GOALS FOR TREATMENT BEFORE BEGINNING MASSAGE

Setting goals for the treatment plan allows the practitioner to inform the client of what the expectations are for treatment. Both long-term and short-term goals can be set based on the condition of the client and the expectations for treatment. Setting goals allows the practitioner to map out a proper treatment plan that will best achieve those goals and gives the practitioner measurable data with which to evaluate the treatment plan for effectiveness. A client who knows and understands both the long-term and short-term goals will better acknowledge the need to be patient in seeing results and is more likely to feel motivated towards achieving those goals. It is important that the practitioner set realistic goals that can be achieved so that the client is seeing continuous improvement and is more apt to work towards the goals. Many times, clients will have unrealistic expectations regarding the effectiveness of the treatment. A practitioner who makes the goals very clear is more likely to develop strong and lasting relationships with clients.

INVOLVING THE CLIENT IN SETTING GOALS FOR TREATMENT

A practitioner should be setting both long-term and short-term goals with each client. A long-term goal may be a few weeks from the first session, or it could be longer if the client has more severe issues to work with. A short-term goal could be a goal for the current session or the week, depending on the length of the treatment plan. When the practitioner involves the client in this goal setting, it assists in the success of the treatment in several ways. By thoroughly explaining the goals to a client, the practitioner can be sure that informed consent has been received and the client is prepared to begin the treatment plan. Setting goals with the client will also give motivation to the client. It gives the client a purpose and a feeling of engagement and ownership in their own wellness. Setting goals also gives measurable and realistic expectations of the treatment plan outcome. This prevents the client from having unrealistic expectations of how massage can help improve the condition. When a practitioner takes the time to explain the treatment goals, this also will build trust between the practitioner and the client, which makes the therapeutic relationship stronger.

PAIN SCALE AND EVALUATION OF CLIENT'S RESPONSE TO PREVIOUS TREATMENTS

The pain scale is a number, usually from 1 to 10, that defines the client's current pain level. 1 would be little or no pain. 10 would be extreme pain. Establishing the level of pain during the initial consultation is critical to understanding the client's pain and giving a reference point to look for improvement. After establishing the initial pain scale, the practitioner should ask for the client's pain level at the end of the first session and before and after each subsequent session. If the treatment is effective, the practitioner should see an overall downward trend of the pain scale number. If the client is reporting increased pain levels, or if the levels are remaining constant, then the practitioner will need to reevaluate the treatment plan for effectiveness. It would be normal for the client to have days where the pain may be slightly higher from the last session, but the overall trend should be for the pain scale number to decrease. Depending on the severity of the condition, the goal may be to lower the pain scale number significantly or to achieve a pain level of 0.

CLIENT REPORTING NO IMPROVEMENT AFTER 6 WEEKS OF WEEKLY MASSAGE

A client who has been receiving massage for six weeks should be seeing improvement in their condition. If not, the practitioner should step back and review the treatment plan and further interview the client to inquire about other factors which may be affecting the outcome. If a client has a chronic condition, results can be small and incremental. However, six weeks should be long enough to expect to see some form of improvement in the condition. If this is not happening, the therapist needs to ask the client about other factors that may be affecting the outcome, such as stress, medications, other illnesses, and activities. If the practitioner can find no other factors that could be affecting the symptoms, then a full evaluation of the treatment plan should be done. The practitioner may not be using the most effective techniques, or the level or frequency of treatment may be inadequate or too much. Reaching out to colleagues who have treated this type of condition can be helpful. The client may also require a referral to a medical professional if one has not previously been made. It is possible that other medical interventions may be needed.

TREATMENT PLAN

A treatment plan is a plan agreed upon by the client and practitioner. It lays out a map of what types of massage techniques can and should be used and what the goals of those techniques are. The treatment plan should include plans for each individual session as well as an overall plan. The treatment plan should be defined by measurable and realistic goals and the client should clearly understand what is going to happen. It is important that it be adaptable in order to make adjustments for treatments that are not proving effective. Information that has been learned in the intake, medical history forms, and interview should be used to develop the treatment plan. The client's preferences and needs should be taken into account and all indications and contraindications should be considered. It is important to prioritize what the client feels is most important. All information should be reviewed with the client and consent given before beginning treatment.

IMPORTANCE OF UNDERSTANDING REFLEX AND MECHANICAL EFFECTS OF MASSAGE TECHNIQUES

Mechanical effects are the direct effects that the massage has on the tissues the practitioner is in contact with. Reflex effects are responses that occur indirectly to touch and are created through the nervous or energy systems of the body. Before a practitioner begins a massage treatment, it is important to understand the effects that each technique produces. Massage affects muscles, lymph, blood circulation, the nervous system, and the skin. Being aware of these effects can prevent the practitioner from causing harm. For example, if a client is at risk of blood clots, applying effleurage to the legs could cause a blood clot to loosen and move to the lungs, causing a pulmonary embolism, which could be fatal. It is also important for a practitioner to understand contraindications and how they apply to massage techniques. Certain techniques could be contraindicated for specific conditions. Having a good understanding of the reflex and mechanical effects of massage will also allow the practitioner to give the client the most effective and enjoyable massage possible and increase the likelihood of achieving the results laid out in the treatment plan.

Ethics, Boundaries, Laws, and Regulations

Ethical Behavior

SETTING AND MAINTAINING PROFESSIONAL BOUNDARIES

Setting appropriate professional boundaries is critical for the massage practitioner because massage therapy is a field in which boundaries can be easily crossed due to the personal nature of the service being offered. These boundaries should be outlined in the policies and procedures of the practice and given to the client at the time of the first appointment. This will provide a framework for the professional relationship between the client and the practitioner. The practitioner can maintain these boundaries by being very clear with the client what the boundaries are and following them strictly in all interactions. This covers such things as how much personal information the therapist shares with the client, starting and ending the massage sessions on time, and being very clear about the fee and how and when payment will be accepted. Once a practitioner does not stay within one of these preset boundaries, it opens the door for inappropriate and even unlawful behavior to occur.

ACCOUNTABILITY

A massage therapist must demonstrate accountability, the ability to take on the responsibilities of a professional. Being accountable means taking responsibility when massage therapy produces an adverse reaction, as well as taking credit for the positive consequences of therapy. In order to be truly accountable, one needs to fully understand the scope of the practice of massage therapy, as well as the code of ethics that must be followed by professionals. Only by understanding the rules of professional practice and the limitations on a massage therapist can one truly take responsibility and be accountable.

HANDLING ETHICAL ISSUES AT WORK

Sooner or later, you will be required to resolve an ethical issue in your professional practice. This issue may or may not have arisen because of your own conduct. Nevertheless, it is your responsibility as an ethical professional to do everything within your power to resolve the issue. First, you should gather as much information as you need to make an informed decision. You should then determine who will be affected by your decision. If necessary, you should contact relevant law enforcement authorities. You may also find it helpful to consult the code of ethics for your jurisdiction. Finally, you should make what you consider to be the ethical decision, and then explain your decision and its consequences to all relevant parties.

Professional Boundaries

IMPORTANCE OF MAINTAINING BOUNDARIES

Boundaries are defined as the personal comfort zones that each person maintains for his own security. Boundaries are intangible and unseen. The acceptable distance from one person's body to another individual varies, and is dependent on each individual's personal preferences. Boundaries can be divided into four types: physical, emotional, intellectual, and sexual. They serve as a personal protective device and, during the course of the massage, the practitioner should be aware of any subtle nuances that would let him know that the client may be on the verge of discomfort. It is important that the practitioner be aware of the client's boundaries, and vital that they exhibit the utmost respect, concern, and professionalism at all times.

TYPES OF PROFESSIONAL BOUNDARIES

There are eight issues related to professional boundaries. They include:

1. **Language**- The choice of words, tone, phrasing, and intonation help to create a safe, secure, peaceful environment.
2. **Touch** – Touch during a massage is necessary. However, skin-to-skin contact should only occur at the parts of the body that are being massaged. The genital area is to be avoided, and draping should be provided for all areas not being massaged.
3. **Time** – Adherence to set appointment times shows respect for the client's time and other personal activities. Also, open communication regarding policies for missed appointments, no shows, and lateness helps to define the boundaries between the client and the practitioner.
4. **Money** – Defining the fee schedule for services rendered in advance of the therapeutic sessions helps to define boundaries. Charging various fees based on a person's skin color, gender, relationship status, etc. does not reflect the type of professionalism all healthcare professionals should be trying to achieve.
5. **Location of services received** – This refers to the location at which massage services are received. Boundaries are less likely to be crossed when the client's safety, comfort, and security are taken into consideration.
6. **Interpersonal space** – This refers to the distance between the practitioner and the client. For sensitive individuals, it is one of the boundaries crossed most frequently.
7. **Appearance** – The impression the massage therapist practitioner makes on their clients is influenced by their appearance. Good hygiene and modest clothing promote a sense of professionalism.
8. **Self-disclosure** – Any personal information provided by the client to the practitioner should be directly related to the treatment and therapy at hand.

Code of Ethics Violations

CODE OF ETHICS

A code of ethics defines the roles and responsibilities assigned to the members of a given profession. Many of the professional organizations for massage therapists have issued codes of ethics. These codes are all somewhat different, but contain a few common elements. Massage therapists are required to strive to provide the best service to their clients, but to never administer treatment for which they have not been trained. Massage therapists are forbidden from practicing any form of discrimination when they deal with clients. They are required to obey all of the laws in their jurisdiction, and to accept responsibility for their actions. They are required to act professionally at all times, and to avoid conflicts of interest and unprofessional relationships with clients.

> **Review Video: Ethical and Professional Standards**
> Visit mometrix.com/academy and enter code: 391843

The Therapeutic Relationship

NATURE OF THE THERAPEUTIC RELATIONSHIP

The relationship between a massage therapist and his or her clients is often described as a therapeutic relationship, one in which one person is responsible for improving the health and quality of life of another person in exchange for money. There is a subtle dynamic at work in this

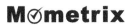

relationship, however, and therapists need to be aware of this. For one thing, it is essential to note that the client is in a significantly weaker position in the relationship. He or she is unlikely to know much about the treatment, will be placed in various compromising positions throughout the therapy, and will have to rely on the professionalism and efficacy of the therapist. The therapist should be conscious of the fact that the client has placed him or herself in a vulnerable position voluntarily, and should make sure that the client's trust has been well placed. The therapist is responsible for upholding the highest professional standards and not taking advantage of the power he or she holds over the client.

Dual Relationships

DUAL RELATIONSHIP

A dual relationship occurs when the client and practitioner enter in to a relationship that is secondary to the therapeutic relationship. This can be a social, romantic, or sexual relationship. Sometimes, dual relationships happen because the client and practitioner are part of the same social circle before the therapeutic relationship begins. This can be managed by maintaining confidentiality and professionalism at all times. Problems can occur when a social or romantic relationship grows out of the initial therapeutic relationship. It is against the ethical practices of a massage practitioner to become romantically or sexually involved with a client. This not only complicates the therapeutic relationship but could also raise legal issues for the practitioner. Considering that many romantic or sexual relationships end poorly, this could open the practitioner to accusations of sexual assault or sexual imposition. If a practitioner begins to have feelings for a client, the therapeutic relationship should be ended before a personal relationship begins. If a client begins making advances toward the practitioner, then a strict boundary should be set. At times, it may be best to end the therapeutic relationship to prevent any problems in the future and also for the comfort of both parties involved.

Sexual Misconduct

HANDLING ISSUES RELATED TO SEXUALITY

Massage is a sensual activity, and so a massage therapist needs to be careful to maintain appropriate sexual boundaries during his or her professional work. At no time should a massage therapist come into direct contact with the genitalia of their clients. It is not uncommon for a client to become sexually aroused during the course of a massage. This is only natural, as massage tends to stimulate the parasympathetic nervous system and direct more blood flow to the genitals. One way to deal with this problem is to deliver more rapid, drumming strokes to the body, which tends to stifle arousal. Another strategy is to simply explain to the client the physiological reasons for his or her arousal and leave it at that. It is not considered sexual harassment to simply describe to a client the natural changes that occur during massage, so long as no effort is made to violate the boundary between client and therapist.

Massage/Bodywork-Related Laws and Regulations

ADOPTING A SET OF ETHICAL GUIDELINES AND A PROFESSIONAL SCOPE OF PRACTICE

A massage practitioner who adopts a set of ethical guidelines and a professional scope of practice will find it much easier to navigate ethical and professional dilemmas that will ultimately occur in the course of doing business. By creating these guidelines and standards, the practitioner has strategies to prepare for situations that may be confusing or difficult. Having good ethics means

Ethics, Boundaries, Laws, and Regulations

that the practitioner shows concern for the general public, clients, and the reputation of the business as well as the field of massage. These guidelines will serve to reduce the risk of harm or injury that could occur due to the abuse of power in the therapeutic relationship. This will make the client feel comfortable and the massage more effective. Having a written policy for a professional scope of practice will also make it clear to clients what conditions can and cannot be treated and serve as a reminder to the practitioner that the first priority of treatment is to do no harm. By going outside of the scope of training and ability, the practitioner will put the client at risk and possibly cause damage to the practitioner's reputation.

HIPAA

The Health Insurance Portability and Accountability Act (HIPAA) was enacted by Congress in 1996. It regulates group health plans and certain health insurance policies. HIPAA also covers the privacy of Protected Health Information (PHI). This privacy rule requires that health providers must have written consent before disclosing PHI unless it is for the purpose of treatment, payment, or health care operations. Under HIPAA, it is required that covered providers take necessary steps to protect the privacy of PHI and the confidentiality of communications with individuals. Individuals have the right to request PHI and receive that information within 30 days. An individual who feels that HIPAA is not being upheld can file a complaint with the Department of Health and Human Services and large fines can be leveled. Employees of covered organizations must be trained in HIPAA policy, and proper documentation and records must be maintained in order to remain in compliance.

> **Review Video: HIPAA**
> Visit mometrix.com/academy and enter code: 412009

APPLICATION TO MASSAGE PRACTITIONERS

Covered entities under HIPAA are any health providers who transmit health information to a third party for billing purposes. In general, this will not cover massage practitioners because most do not accept health insurance directly. However, if the massage practitioner is providing services for an entity that would be covered under HIPAA, then certain privacy rules would be required. It is recommended that a massage practitioner who is not sure of their status under HIPAA consult a knowledgeable attorney who can assist with answering questions regarding status and confirm that the practitioner is in compliance. Massage practitioners should always maintain client confidentiality, even when the situation is not covered under HIPAA guidelines. Privacy is only a small part of HIPAA. There are many requirements that must be met under this law. A massage practitioner should be sure to educate themselves fully on the requirements of this law and consult an attorney with any questions.

EDUCATIONAL REQUIREMENTS FOR CERTIFICATION

There are no mandated national educational requirements for certification or licensure as a massage therapist. However, there are certain elements required for certification that are common among all jurisdictions. For instance, almost all states require applicants to have a high school diploma or GED. Most licensing organizations require at least 500 hours of instruction in massage therapy, with emphasis on anatomy, physiology, pathology, modalities of bodywork and massage, contraindications for massage, massage safety, and professional practice. Usually, individuals are required to pass a standardized test in order to receive their license. There are a few different standardized tests used throughout the United States for this purpose.

REVOCATION OR SUSPENSION OF LICENSE

If you violate the code of ethics or regulations set by the governing body, you may have your massage therapist's license revoked or suspended. For instance, if you are convicted of a felony

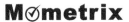

while practicing as a massage therapist, your license may be suspended. The following events can also be cause for the revocation or suspension of a license: prostitution, willful negligence, substance abuse, deceptive advertising, and sexual misconduct in the line of duty. Furthermore, if the organization that issued your license determines that you used deception in order to obtain a license, it may be revoked.

Scope of Practice

SCOPE OF PRACTICE FOR WELLNESS MASSAGE

A scope of practice is the list of activities a given professional has the right to perform under on his or her license. The precise description of a massage therapist's scope of practice is different in every state. It is important for a therapist to understand his or her scope of practice so that he or she does not overstep professional boundaries. The scope of practice for wellness massage is smaller than that for therapeutic massage. This is because the goals of wellness massage are more general and less ambitious. In order to practice wellness massage, a massage therapist must have general training in the anatomy, physiology, pathology, and modalities of wellness massage. He or she is then authorized to use these modalities to promote circulation and reduce stress.

INFORMED CONSENT FORMS

Since the massage therapist understands his or her professional business much better than his or her clients, it is the responsibility of the therapist to describe in detail any proposed treatment before initiation. This is done by means of an informed consent form, in which the proposed treatment is described in full, including any potential risks of the treatment. The presentation of an informed consent document gives the client a chance to ask questions. An informed consent form may also include a list of actions which would result in the immediate termination of treatment; it is a good idea for the therapist to publish such a list in the event that a dispute with the client arises.

HIPPOCRATIC OATH

The Hippocratic Oath first appeared in Greek medical texts in the fifth century BC. Its primary message is to do no harm. This applies to physicians and all medical practitioners, including massage. Some of the key messages in the more modern version of the oath translate very well to the field of massage. One of the tenets of the Hippocratic Oath is to avoid overtreatment. This is an important lesson that massage practitioners need to remember. It is very tempting to use massage as a cure for every ailment or to overdo pressure or the amount of time spent on an area of the body. The Hippocratic Oath also reminds us that medicine is an art and that warmth, understanding, and compassion are vital to a person's care. These are essential aspects of massage. A very important part of the Hippocratic Oath that should be observed by massage practitioners is the concept of not being afraid to say, "I know not." It is extremely important that massage practitioners understand when to refer a client to a more appropriate medical professional and respect the limits of what massage can do to relieve pain or disease.

PERFORMING A TECHNIQUE WITHOUT TRAINING

Massage has many effects on the systems of the body. When a practitioner performs a technique in which they are not trained, it could prove harmful to the client. Massage techniques are designed to create specific physiological effects on the body. A practitioner who has not been trained in a technique may not understand the contraindications or how it may affect a client physiologically. Most techniques also require a certain level of skill in order to use the appropriate pressure and pace. Applying a technique too vigorously could cause pain or injury to the client. Certain techniques, such as stretching and joint movements, require more skill, especially when working

Ethics, Boundaries, Laws, and Regulations

129

with older or frail clients. A practitioner who is not trained in using these types of techniques could cause injuries such as dislocations or bone fractures if the patient is not able to tolerate the movements. Certain techniques may also have absolute contraindications for specific medical conditions, so it is important that a practitioner understand when and when not to use specific techniques.

TREATING A CLIENT WHO HAS STOPPED MEDICATION TO TRY HOLISTIC THERAPIES

A new client reports that they have a serious, chronic medical condition and have stopped taking their medications in order to try more holistic therapies. The practitioner knows that massage is indicated for this condition but is aware that massage alone cannot resolve this condition.

In this situation, it would be acceptable for the massage practitioner to offer treatment because massage is indicated for this condition. However, ethically speaking, it is important that the practitioner emphasize to the client that massage is not a cure for this chronic condition, and it is recommended that the client consult with a physician in order to discuss treatment options and any risks involved in stopping a medication. It is also important that the practitioner monitor the client's condition during future sessions in case there is a change in overall health. The practitioner is not doing harm by treating the individual if massage is advised but must take the client's overall well-being into consideration during all treatments. If the practitioner knows of a holistic physician that would be beneficial to this client, then a referral can be made.

REQUESTS FOR SPORTS MASSAGE WHEN NOT TRAINED IN SPORTS MASSAGE

Sports massage generally consists of a variety of techniques such as myofascial release, neuromuscular therapy, and stretching and deep tissue massage. If the practitioner is not specifically trained in sports massage, but has knowledge and training in the aforementioned techniques, then it would be acceptable to perform those techniques on a client who has requested a sports massage session. The practitioner should inform the client that they do not have sports massage training but are capable of performing techniques that are beneficial to the athlete. At this point, the client could choose to deny the service and seek out a practitioner who is trained in sports massage. If a practitioner is receiving many requests from clients for a particular modality, then it would be recommended that the practitioner seek training in that particular modality in order to offer better service to their clientele. If a practitioner does not have training in any of the techniques used in sports massage, then the practitioner should inform the client. The client may choose to accept a massage that is not a sports massage in order to receive general benefits.

Professional Communication

PROFESSIONAL COMMUNICATION SKILLS

One of the most important but least talked about aspects of ethical professional practice as a massage therapist is effective communication. In order to serve a client, the therapist needs to be able to describe his or her work and understand the concerns, complaints, and questions of the client. The therapist needs to establish a relationship with the client in which the client feels comfortable making requests and offering constructive criticism. Too often, massage therapists cultivate their reputations as experts to such a degree that a client does not feel comfortable asking for what he or she wants. In order to effectively serve his or her clients, a therapist needs to be able to listen without judgment. Furthermore, the client's goals should always be the primary consideration when the therapist is making decisions.

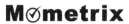

ASKING SPECIFIC QUESTIONS DURING CLIENT CONSULTATIONS

The initial consultation is perhaps the most important session in any therapeutic story because it establishes the relationship between the therapist and the client. In order to get the most out of this and any subsequent consultations, a therapist needs to be able to ask pertinent and effective questions. It is important for the therapist to establish an environment in which the client feels comfortable discussing his or her health. The therapist should remember that many clients will not have a vocabulary for what they are trying to express, and so the therapist should help draw their feelings out without dominating the conversation or distorting the client's point of view. A therapist should ask questions which give the client a chance to ruminate on his or her health history, and should seek to clarify any uncertain points by asking specific, objective questions.

NONVERBAL COMMUNICATION

Because massage therapy is a profession concerned with touch, it is not surprising that some of the most important communication between massage therapists and clients is nonverbal. Nonverbal communication is not limited to touch, however. In order to establish a positive working relationship with a client, a massage therapist needs to communicate warmth and accessibility with his or her body language. A smile and a relaxed posture can be contagious, and can help a client derive extra benefits from a massage session. Also, a therapist needs to consider the body language of a client, and should tread lightly when a client seems peevish or defensive. Additionally, a client's body language will sometimes give the therapist information about his or her condition that the client cannot express through words.

Confidentiality

CONFIDENTIALITY

A massage therapist is required to respect the privacy of his or her clients by maintaining strict confidentiality standards. This means keeping client records in a secure location, and not sharing them with other practitioners without the permission of the client. In order to provide health information to another professional, even the client's doctor, you must receive permission from the client. Confidentiality can only be violated when it is obvious that there is an immediate danger to the client or some other person. In some rare cases, a client may not want to be recognized outside of the therapy environment. If you are in public and notice that a client seems to be avoiding you, do not make special efforts to attract the attention of the client.

Ethics, Boundaries, Laws, and Regulations

Guidelines for Professional Practice

Proper and Safe Use of Equipment

TYPICAL SET-UP FOR A MASSAGE THERAPY PRACTICE

Depending on the extent of the practice and the funds available, the therapist should have basic equipment for the following areas of the practice: the office area, the massage area, and the restroom facility or hydrotherapy area. An independent massage therapist with a smaller practice will generally work out of their home or a small office. The business area should be cordoned off from clients for confidentiality purposes and to allow for privacy during client consultations. The restroom facility provides a place for clients to shower before and after the massage, and is also a place for the massage therapist to wash his or her hands between each massage. Finally, the massage area is made up of the massage table, a stool, a storage area for linens, oils, creams, etc., and a dressing area for the client. Pillows or bolsters should be readily available to help make the client more comfortable during the massage. Appropriate drapes should be located nearby to give clients privacy during the massage.

APPROPRIATE MASSAGE ROOM SIZE, TEMPERATURE, AND FURNISHINGS

A typical massage room should be no less than 10 feet wide by 12 feet long in order to accommodate the massage table, desk, and storage areas for linens and lotions, and to provide enough space for the therapist to adequately maneuver around the table to perform the massage. Considering that the client will not have clothes on during the massage, it is important to keep the room at an ideal temperature to prevent chills. A temperature of 72° Fahrenheit would ensure the comfort of the client as well as the therapist, who may become overheated while performing the massage.

APPROPRIATE MASSAGE ROOM VENTILATION, LIGHTING, AND MUSIC

In order to help their clients relax, massage therapists need to make some environmental adjustments to the massage room. Proper ventilation should be in place to provide fresh air that is free from odors. The lighting in the room should not be harsh and glaring; it should be reflective or soft, which will make the client feel comfortable. Purchasing dimmer switches to adjust lighting according to the client's needs and preferences would be a simple and worthwhile investment. Music also helps to promote relaxation; however, it is best to make music selections based on the client's preferences rather than the therapist's.

APPROPRIATE MASSAGE TABLE HEIGHT

Next to the massage therapist's hands, a massage table is one of the most important pieces of equipment. It should be determined whether the table will be used in a home setting or in an office environment. The table should be firm, stable, and comfortable for the client. A table that is an appropriate height is one that enables the therapist to place his hands flat on the surface while keeping his arms straight. This is the best height to provide leverage and help prevent fatigue of the back, neck, shoulders, and arms while performing the massage.

APPROPRIATE MASSAGE TABLE SIZE AND PADDING

Many tables are made with hydraulic or manual height adjustments, which are especially useful if different therapists will be using the same table. The standard size of a massage table is approximately 29 inches wide by 68 to 72 inches long. This can accommodate most average-sized clients, but may be too short for taller individuals. The table's padding should consist of at least one

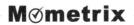

Guidelines for Professional Practice

to two inches of high-density foam for optimal comfort for the client. A vinyl covering is preferred over any other type of covering, due to ease of cleaning and sanitizing between clients. To care for vinyl, a solution of mild detergent is all that is needed. Some massage tables are also adjustable to accommodate patients with different needs.

Therapist Hygiene

APPROPRIATE HYGIENE REGIMEN FOR A MASSAGE THERAPIST

In order to prevent infection and the spread of disease, a massage therapist needs to engage in a comprehensive hygiene regimen. The most important part of this regimen is handwashing after every client encounter. During handwashing, an antibacterial soap should be used. All jewelry should be removed from the hands. Alcohol-based hand sanitizers are an acceptable alternative. A therapist should also put on latex gloves whenever he or she is required to clean up the bodily fluids of a client. A therapist should clean his or her equipment regularly with antiseptics, and should occasionally use a stronger disinfectant, making sure to rinse the equipment thoroughly with warm water afterwards.

MODES OF INFECTION

Massage therapy can be a breeding ground for infection if the massage therapist is not careful. To maintain their clientele, a therapist must have a facility that is clean and sterile, and must protect against the spread of disease to safeguard the well-being of their clients. Following strict laws regulating sanitation procedures, the massage therapist must utilize disinfectants, antiseptics, and other cleaning agents to maintain a healthy environment. Illness- and disease-causing pathogens are transmitted from one infected person to another directly or indirectly. They can enter the body through inhalation, ingestion, broken skin, contact with mucous membranes, or sexual contact.

Sanitation and Cleanliness

TRANSMISSION OF PATHOGENS, BACTERIA, VIRUSES, AND FUNGI

Pathogens can be transmitted through beverages or food. Types of pathogens the massage therapist should be concerned about are bacteria, fungus, and viruses. Bacteria are most commonly found on dirty surfaces and in unclean water, and can cause illnesses such as pneumonia, typhoid fever, TB, diphtheria, and syphilis, just to name a few. Viruses can invade living hosts and transmit diseases such as colds, mumps, measles, and pneumonia. Warm, moist environments create an ideal environment for fungi and mold to reproduce. Fungal infections are responsible for ringworm, athlete's foot, and Candida.

UNIVERSAL PRECAUTIONS TO PROTECT INDIVIDUALS FROM CONTAMINATION

The following steps are considered necessary precautions to stop the spread of infection:

- Washing hands with soap and water before and after contact with each client
- Using disposable paper towels rather than cloth
- Washing skin and hands thoroughly if any contact is made with contaminated fluids
- Wearing gloves when performing certain tasks and washing hands after removing the gloves
- Washing any linens contaminated with blood or bodily fluids in hot water with bleach and drying them in a hot dryer

- Handling contaminated linens as little as possible and separating them from other linens
- Cleaning surfaces such as walls and ceilings with disinfectant if they come in contact with spills requiring sanitation

Safety Practices

MAINTENANCE OF SAFE MASSAGE THERAPY FACILITIES

When we think of safety in the context of massage therapy, we usually think of the physical manipulations, which have the potential to stress and strain the body of the client or the therapist. However, it is equally important for the facilities at the massage therapist's office to be safe. By facilities, we mean all of the buildings, furnishings, and equipment used by the massage therapist and his or her customers. In order to maintain a high level of safety, a massage therapist needs to keep the buildings clean, uncluttered, well-lit, and sanitized. All equipment should be checked frequently to make sure it is sturdy and safe for use. Every massage office should have an accessible first-aid kit and the phone numbers for emergency services posted next to the telephone.

MAINTAINING THERAPIST SAFETY

Although a massage therapist primarily focuses on improving the quality of life of his or her clients, the therapist also needs to protect him or herself from injury or illness. To this end, the therapist should wash his or her hands after every encounter with a client. The therapist should not perform any therapies that are outside his or her scope of expertise, and should be aware of any counterindications for massage practice. In order to reduce the risk of infection in the massage environment, the therapist should clean and sterilize equipment with a disinfectant regularly. The therapist should also ensure that his or her work environment has adequate ventilation.

MAINTAINING CLIENT SAFETY

The best way to maintain client safety is to have clean and safe facilities, and to communicate any potential hazards to the client. For instance, clients should be alerted whenever the therapist is about to position his or her body in a potentially stressful manner. Disabled or elderly clients should be assisted into position, and should also be helped on and off the massage table. Clients who are ill, injured, or have severe allergies should have these conditions thoroughly examined before undergoing massage therapy. In addition, a massage therapist needs to keep a fully-stocked first-aid kit on hand at all times in case the client should suffer some injury. In order to minimize the risk of infection, the massage therapist should wash his or her hands after every client.

Therapist Care

IMPORTANCE OF MASSAGE THERAPIST TAKING GOOD PHYSICAL CARE OF HIS OR HER OWN BODY

A person considering massage therapy should understand that this profession requires a great deal of physical strength. To assist others through massage, the therapist places considerable stress on his own body, which can be injured if proper procedures are not followed when performing the massage on a client. Proper stances, exercises for the hands, and good body mechanics will help eliminate some of the stress on the practitioner. It is important to develop good posture, coordination, balance, and stamina to provide the best possible massages for the client with minimal damage to oneself. As the hands are the most important of the practitioner's tools, flexibility is key to controlling the speed of the massage and pressure sensitivity, along with the ability to conform to the contours of the client's body. Along with proper physical conditioning, the

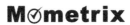

therapist should also concentrate on his emotional state during the massage and not let outside influences mar the session.

LEVERAGE

In order to avoid injury and unnecessary strain on the body, a massage therapist needs to learn proper body mechanics. One of the main principles of body mechanics as it applies to massage therapy is leverage, the technique of producing the greatest amount of pressure on the client with the least amount of work. Basically, leverage is achieved in massage therapy by locking the arms at the elbows and leaning on the client so that the weight of the therapist is doing most of the work. Also, massage therapists should try to stand as close to their clients as possible, as proximity makes the work of creating pressure easier. In order to deliver effective force with the use of leverage, it is important for the massage table to be set low enough that the therapist can lean into the patient without his or her arm being at too much of an angle with his or her torso.

SYMMETRIC AND ASYMMETRIC STANCE

In order to avoid being injured as a result of the repetitive stresses associated with practicing massage therapy, one needs to learn the appropriate uses of the symmetric and asymmetric stances. In the symmetric stance, the feet are shoulder-width apart, with the knees flexed to the same degree and the toes pointed forward. This stance is appropriate when the client is directly in front of the therapist, as the weight is evenly distributed between the legs. In the asymmetric stance, on the other hand, one foot is in front of the other, with the front foot pointed forward and the back foot pointed slightly to the outside. In this pose, the majority of the weight is on the back foot. This stance is appropriate when the therapist is trying to get extra leverage to apply more pressure to the client's body. A massage therapist needs to be able to work comfortably with either the right or left foot forward in the asymmetric stance.

DANGERS OF POOR BODY MECHANICS FOR MASSAGE THERAPISTS

Although massage therapy is primarily a gentle discipline, the repetitive movements and application of pressure can result in injury for therapists with poor body mechanics. In particular, the hands, wrists, and elbows are subject to a great deal of strain during massage. In order to avoid repetitive stress injuries, a therapist should keep the table at the appropriate height (such that the arms are almost fully extended when laid on the client) and avoid applying pressure with too great of an angle from the body. The therapist's back should be kept straight as much as possible, and his or her shoulders should remain back rather than hunched forward. Therapists should also slightly flex their knees, and should be wearing shoes that distribute their weight evenly throughout the foot.

UNIVERSAL PRECAUTIONS PERTAINING TO WEARING OF GLOVES

Universal precautions is a system used to avoid infection caused by exposure to blood and/or bloody body fluids. In this system, all body fluids are assumed to be potentially infectious with a blood-borne pathogen. Examples of blood-borne pathogens are diseases such as HIV and hepatitis. The guidelines for wearing gloves, as it pertains to massage, involve protecting both the practitioner and the client from exposure and ensuring that any soiled massage linens are handled properly. If, at any time, the practitioner's skin is not intact due to injury or any other skin conditions, then gloves must be worn to protect the client. If there are any lesions or weeping dermatitis, then the practitioner must refrain from doing massage until the condition is no longer present. If there is any potential for the practitioner to come into contact with bodily fluids during the massage, then the practitioner should wear gloves. This would include any sores, lesions, or any seeping wounds. Gloves should be disposed of after the massage. Gloves should be worn when

135

handling any items that may have come into contact with blood or other body fluids. Hands should be washed as soon as the gloves are removed.

WEARING A MASK DURING A MASSAGE SESSION

Wearing a mask during a massage session is more often used to protect the client rather than the practitioner. A practitioner may choose to wear a mask if there are upper respiratory symptoms present, such as cough or nasal congestion and drainage. If the practitioner is considered contagious or has a fever, then massage should be refrained from until symptoms have abated. If there is no fever present and the practitioner is known to be no longer contagious, it is acceptable to do massage with a mask to prevent dripping from the mucous membranes and to protect the client and provide comfort from coughing. The practitioner may also choose to wear a mask if the client is immune compromised. A client who is undergoing treatments for cancer or other diseases which may weaken the immune system are at higher risk of exposure to illnesses than non-immune compromised clients. If the practitioner has not felt well or has been exposed to others who are ill, then wearing a mask would be an appropriate safety precaution in order to protect the client from possible exposure.

Draping

PURPOSE OF DRAPING

In order to preserve a client's privacy during massage, a massage therapist will drape the client's body with linens. Besides preventing embarrassment on the part of the client, draping also keeps the client warm, which improves the efficacy of massage. When performing a full body massage, the massage therapist will have to uncover and recover body parts in order to gain access to all the necessary areas. Although the precise requirements for draping vary from state to state, as a general rule, the breasts, genitals, and gluteal cleft should remain covered at all times. The most common form of draping is known as two-sheet draping; it requires one sheet to cover the massage table and another to cover the client. Some more advanced forms of draping may require additional, smaller sheets.

TOP COVER METHOD OF DRAPING

One of the more common styles of draping is known as top cover (or two-sheet) draping. It requires the use of two large sheets: one to cover the massage table, and one large enough to cover the entire client. A set of quality twin bed sheets would be suitable. In a pinch, you can use a couple of large bath towels in place of the top sheet. The patient can be wrapped in the top sheet on the way from the dressing room to the massage table. One of the benefits of a large top sheet is that you can easily lift it up to block your own view, which will allow the client to maneuver into position for the next part of the massage.

TECHNIQUES

At the beginning of the massage, the top cover should be positioned long-ways so that only the client's head is exposed. To massage the torso of a male, simply fold the top cover down to the waist. To massage the arms, simply fold the top cover under the client's arms at the armpits. To massage the torso of a woman, place a towel or pillowcase over the breasts and slide the cover out from under it. To massage a leg, simply slide the top cover back so that only that leg is exposed. When it is time for the client to roll over, you can either hold the cover up to block your view or hold the cover in place while the client rolls beneath it.

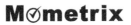

FULL-SHEET METHOD OF DRAPING

Some massage therapists employ the full-sheet method of draping, in which only one large sheet is used to cover both the massage table and the client. A queen-size bed sheet is usually sufficient for this kind of draping. The sheet is placed on the massage table and then folded over the client. It will be necessary to give the client a separate wrap to wear from the dressing room to the massage table. Once the client has been positioned inside the full sheet, the wrap can be removed. Some massage therapists will then take the wrap and lay it across the client's chest in order to hold the full sheet in place.

TECHNIQUES

When a client has been draped according to the full-sheet method of draping, his or her arms can be massaged by discreetly sliding them out from under the top of the sheet. When they are not exposed, the client's arms should be placed at his or her sides underneath the sheet. The legs should be undraped from the foot upwards. Otherwise, the drapes on each leg should be tucked under the legs to prevent the drape from sliding off. To massage the torso of a male, fold the top cover down to the uppermost part of the pubic bone. To massage the torso of a female, place the wrap on top of the breasts and slide the top cover out from under it while the client holds the wrap in place. When the client needs to roll over, only cover him or her from the neck to the knees, and hold the cover in place during the operation.

APPROPRIATE COMMUNICATION DURING THE DRAPING PROCESS

The art of draping a client during massage is somewhat complex, and may make a shy client uneasy. In order to reduce client anxiety, it is a good idea to maintain appropriate communication regarding the purpose of your draping movements. You should explain the intention of draping to every new client before beginning the massage. Before uncovering any part of the client's body, describe what you are about to do. Sometimes, you will need to hold up the sheet to block your own view as the client gets into a different position. You should always remind the client that you will not be able to see them, and then describe the position you would like them to assume. Always give the client an opportunity to ask questions.

Business Practices

TAX STATUS FOR SOLE PROPRIETORSHIP, LLC, AND CORPORATION

SOLE PROPRIETORSHIP

This type of business has one individual owner who is responsible for all expenses, liabilities, and assets. All profits from the business would go to the sole proprietor and that person would be responsible for any losses. For tax purposes, the sole proprietor and the business are considered the same entity. All profits and losses from the business flow through to the owner and are taxed as income. There are also self-employment taxes which must be paid.

LLC

An LLC is a limited liability company. This type of business is a legal entity that allows some of the benefits of a corporation, but with much less paperwork. All profits and losses from this type of business go to the owners and are reported on their individual tax returns. There is not a separate return filed for the business.

CORPORATION

A corporation is a separate business entity from the owners and is subject to regulation and taxation. A charter must be obtained and management of the corporation would be the responsibility of a board of directors. The corporation will file a tax return and pay taxes on profits. Employees will be paid a salary, then pay individual taxes on that salary.

ADVANTAGES AND DISADVANTAGES OF BEING SELF-EMPLOYED AS A MASSAGE THERAPIST

One of the first decisions that must be made after being certified as a massage therapist is whether to go into business for oneself or work as an employee at a spa, doctor's office, or medical facility. There are pros and cons to each situation. Working as a self-employed massage therapist forces the practitioner to be responsible for paying his own employment taxes, paying for needed supplies (such as office equipment and the massage table), and assuming any rental costs for the facility. Disadvantages include the lack of a formal support team, being responsible for managing the paperwork for the business side as a self-employed entity, and the lack of a steady paycheck due to the time needed to build the business. Working in an established environment allows the therapist to have a built-in clientele, without incurring the overhead costs of doing business. Additionally, the therapist has the support of fellow employees to help with increased client loads. The company would also provide benefits such as vacation, sick leave, and health insurance, and would be responsible for paying any state and federal employer taxes.

SOLE PROPRIETORSHIP

A massage therapist has the option of registering their business as a sole proprietor, partnership, limited liability corporation, or corporation. There are advantages and disadvantages to each of these arrangements. A sole proprietorship is a business in which the owner assumes all responsibility for the business, whether from a financial or obligatory standpoint. The individual is also legally responsible for all failures of the business, and may be held accountable if any lawsuits are brought against the company. The courts will see the individual and the business as one entity. Therefore, the person is held legally responsible for any business debt. An advantage of a sole proprietorship is that the owner is not accountable to a board or group of shareholders.

PARTNERSHIP, LIMITED LIABILITY CORPORATION, AND CORPORATION

Under a partnership, two or more individuals share in the successes and failures of the business; all partners share equally in the risk. It is similar to a sole proprietorship in that the group of owners can be held personally responsible for all activities of the business. A limited liability corporation (LLC) is a combination of a partnership and a corporation. A limited liability corporation has some of the same benefits as a corporation, but there is less paperwork involved. Additionally, an LLC offers more protection of one's personal assets in the event of a lawsuit. Finally, a corporation assigns management of the business to a board of directors who share in the policy development and decision-making processes. Stockholders are financially tied to the success of the company, as they share in any profits that are made.

LIMITED LIABILITY COMPANY

A limited liability company is a legal business entity that offers some of the benefits of being a corporation, but with much less paperwork. In a limited liability company, the owners are a separate entity from the business and are protected from some of the liability of the business. All profits and losses from a limited liability company are divided equally among the owners and recorded on the individual income taxes of the owners. In order to create a limited liability company, the owner or owners must file a form with the state in which the business will be operating. Some states will require that a limited liability company have more than one owner and others will allow a sole proprietorship limited liability company. It is important to research the requirements in the state the company is being established, as there will be different requirements for licensing and establishing the business in each state.

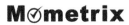

CRITERIA FOR AN INDEPENDENT CONTRACTOR RELATIONSHIP

An independent contractor relationship is defined by the Internal Revenue Service and differentiates the relationship from employment. There are three criteria that need to be met in order to be considered an independent contractor.

1. The independent contractor must have **behavioral control over the work**. This means that the contractor must have control over the hours worked and how the tasks to be done are managed. No specific training and equipment is provided.
2. The independent contractor must have **financial control**. The contractor may pay rent or receive a percentage of fees received. An employee would be paid a salary or hourly wage. Self-employment taxes are the responsibility of the independent contractor.
3. The business relationship must be **independent**. An independent contractor is responsible for all insurance, sick days, and vacation days. The independent contractor is also free to work with other companies. There should be a written agreement explaining how the contractor will provide services and the amount paid for these services.

If these three criteria are not met, then it would be considered an employee relationship and the business owner would be responsible for paying taxes for the employee.

START-UP EXPENSES

The categories of start-up expenses for a business are listed and described below:

- **Rent or lease** – This can include first and last month's rent and deposits for damage
- **Utilities** – Deposits and hook-up charges for all utilities including electric, gas, telephone, and Internet. Some utilities may be paid by landlord.
- **Equipment and supplies** – Massage table, linens, massage oils and lotions, bolsters and pillows, and therapeutic equipment will all be needed to provide services to clients.
- **Furniture** – Office desk and chair, filing cabinet, sound system, chair for clients, lighting and any other miscellaneous furniture needed for comfort of practitioner and clients.
- **Décor** – Pictures, curtains, plants, and accessories will all make the business welcoming for clients.
- **Advertising** – Web site, business cards, flyers or brochures, ads, and signs for building are needed in order to bring in clients.
- **Printing expenses** – Stationery, forms, and other advertising materials will need to be printed professionally.
- **Licenses and permits** – Business license, professional license, and sales tax license will be required.
- **Initial operating expenses** – Opening accounts and covering business expenses until income is sufficient to cover expenses.
- **Professional fees** – Accountant, attorney, web designer and any other professional services that would support the business.
- **Insurance** – Personal and professional liability insurance, health and disability insurance will be needed.

CHOOSING A BUSINESS LOCATION

Choosing the business location is one of the most important decisions that a practitioner can make. It is critical to whether the business will be successful or fail. The site should meet all of the needs of the business, fit the image of the business, and be properly zoned and in a location that will support the business. There must be clientele in the area with the financial means to purchase massage services. The location must also fit the practitioner's budget. If the business is easy to find, especially if it easily visible from the street, it is more likely to attract customers. The ideal location must also have appropriate space to accommodate massage services. There should be room for treatments, a client waiting area, and space for a desk and filing cabinets. It is also important to notice the noise levels in the building and surrounding area. The practitioner should also investigate the area for competition. Too many massage practitioners in one area could mean there won't be enough business or it could mean there is a very high demand in that area. The practitioner can learn more about the area by contacting the local Chamber of Commerce.

MISSION STATEMENT

A mission statement sets the tone for the focus and mission of a business. It should be a general statement that expresses the values of and sets an intention for the business. This statement can be used in marketing and advertising materials and should reflect the image the business wishes to portray. The mission statement should be written with careful consideration because it sets the tone for the business's public image. It should describe the products and services it plans to provide, its primary customers, and what the overall vision is for the business. The mission statement should demonstrate to any party who reads it what the business stands for and what is its mission. It is an opportunity to describe what makes the business unique and why its customers should trust the business to meet their needs. A mission statement does not generally change over time. It should be continuous and consistent.

BUSINESS BOOKKEEPING SYSTEM

A bookkeeping system is a way for a business to track and maintain accurate records. A small business bookkeeping system does not need to be complicated, but it should contain certain elements that will assist the business owner in tracking the progress of the business and meet the requirements for filing taxes and managing any employees. The bookkeeping system must track business income. An income ledger allows the business owner to track all receipts of money received from products and services. It should list the classifications and sources of all income and have a column for sales tax if necessary. All income should be dated. The income ledger can be updated daily or monthly depending on the size of the business. The business must also track all disbursements for expenses. This information can come from the check book or credit card statement. Based on the income coming in and the payments going out, a profit and loss statement can be created to show if the business is profitable or losing money from normal operations. The bookkeeping system should also track accounts receivable, which is money owed to the business; as well as accounts payable, which is money the business owes.

APPOINTMENT BOOK

An appointment book is an important part of a successful massage business. Managing appointments ensures that the practitioner does not miss an appointment or book more than one client at any time. It also assists in time management. It is critical for a massage practitioner to be on time to appointments and allow sufficient time between clients so as not to be rushed or allow the day to become behind schedule. A well-organized appointment book will have space for the client's name, phone number, and an address if the practitioner is doing an outcall. The appointment book can be paper-based or electronic, depending on the type of business and the practitioner's preferences. If the practitioner is traveling regularly, an appointment book that is portable would be necessary. If two different books are being used for travel and office, the practitioner should be sure to consolidate the two to avoid double booking. It is also important to maintain client's confidentiality. An appointment book can also serve as a file to maintain records for mileage and business expenses.

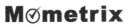

INCOME OR PROFIT AND LOSS STATEMENT

An income or profit and loss statement provides a summary of the profits and losses that a business has incurred during a set period of time. The income statement can be done monthly, quarterly, or annually. The profit and loss or income statement is an excellent tool for the business owner to compare profits or losses in one period to the profits or losses in another period. This can show the health of the business and allow the owner to make adjustments as needed to increase revenue or decrease expenditures. To prepare a profit and loss or income statement, the business owner will need a register of all income sources within the time period being analyzed and calculate a total of all the revenues. A listing of all disbursements would also need to be totaled to determine the amount of expenses incurred during the period. Once both income and expenses have been calculated, the total expenses are subtracted from the total revenues, and this will give the amount of the profit or loss.

TARGET MARKET

A target market is defined as a group of the population that has similar characteristics that the business owner would like to attract to the business's services. Choosing a target market allows the business owner to personalize advertising and marketing activities in order to attract that particular population group. There can be any number of parameters for choosing a target market. It can be very specific or very broad. Some of the parameters that can define a target market are age, gender, income, location, occupation, or recreational activities and interests. A massage practitioner can choose a target market in more than one way. A new business can look at the demographics of an area and the types of activities and occupations that are common and develop the business to serve that market. A target market can also be chosen based on the practitioner's skills and interests. If sports massage is the practitioner's strength, then athletes would be the target market. If the business is already established but looking to expand, the practitioner could look through client files to find common factors, then target new marketing and advertising to that market.

BUSINESS PROMOTION

The objective to promoting a business is to be visible in the community and become known. Promotion also will create a feeling of desire among potential customers to use the product or service. Here are some common methods of business promotion.

- **Developing promotional materials** – This would include business cards, brochures, stationery, and newsletters.
- **Internet marketing** – Having a website is important for a business owner to communicate information to clients or potential clients. Using email is also an excellent way for a business owner to stay in contact with clients.
- **Advertising** – Magazine and newspaper ads and listings, signs, or giveaways like pens and calendars are great ways to advertise a business.
- **Public relations** – Writing articles for magazines or newspapers or speaking to groups allows the business to be seen by a large number of people.
- **Encouraging referrals** – Asking current clients to refer friends and family and even offering incentive discounts for doing so is an easy way to build business.
- **Client retention** – It is six times more expensive to obtain new clients than it is to retain current ones. Engaging with clients and encouraging them to return with excellent customer service is a way to maintain income without further investing in the business.

Guidelines for Professional Practice

141

HIRING NEW EMPLOYEES

As the massage therapy practice grows, it may become necessary to add to one's staff to serve more clients. Some businesses hire massage therapists as independent contractors, while others hire them as full-time employees. As an independent contractor, the practitioner is responsible for paying his own taxes, and will need to file tax forms 1099 and 1096 if he exceeds $600.00 in income during the previous year. As a full-time employee, the employer is responsible for providing an hourly paycheck and a benefits package. In either case, the person hired can help the business succeed or fail, depending on his professionalism and how personable he or she is with clients. When seeking out new employees, it is important to verify all credentials and licensing, ensure that appropriate training is provided, and work with the person to help him achieve the business's goals.

QUESTIONS NOT ALLOWED DURING INTERVIEW PROCESS

If a massage practitioner plans to hire employees to work for the business, it is important to have an understanding of the types of questions that cannot be asked during an interview. Certain questions are considered discriminatory and must be avoided. An interviewer cannot ask candidates how old they are, but it is acceptable to ask if the candidate is over 18 years of age. Asking the candidate about race, religion, or nation of origin is not acceptable as well. The interviewer may not inquire if the candidate has children or plans to have them in the future. Any questions pertaining to political affiliations, sexual orientation, or marital status must be avoided. It would be acceptable for the interviewer to explain the physical demands of the job and inquire if the applicant will be able to complete the tasks required for the position but may not ask about a disability. Questions should be focused on the abilities, background, and experience of the candidate and should stay away from inquiries of a personal nature.

CLIENT FILE

What a practitioner chooses to include in a client file varies by practice. The most common and necessary information would be the client's contact information and emergency contact number. There should also be an intake and health history form, plus the treatment plan and records of individual treatment sessions. The more detailed the information, the more prepared the practitioner will be if the need to contact the client or refer to previous sessions arise. If there has been a referral from another health practitioner, it is important to keep the referral letter in the client file, as well as any other communications to or from referrals. Financial and billing records should also be kept in the file. Any special needs or requests from the client should be kept in the file for future reference. Records should be kept up-to-date so the practitioner can easily access the necessary information quickly and conveniently.

KEEPING TAX-RELATED BUSINESS RECORDS

The IRS has set guidelines for keeping tax related documents, but there is some variation in recommendations about how long records should be kept. The IRS says that records should be kept three years from when the tax return was filed. If the business filed for a loss or a deduction due to bad debt, it is recommended the records be kept for seven years. Most lawyers and accountants would suggest that all records be kept for seven years. Payroll tax records should be kept for at least four years from when the payroll tax has been paid. All employee files and accounting and operational records should be kept for seven years. This would include budgets, check ledgers, profit and loss statements, bank statements, credit card statements, checkbook stubs, and canceled checks. All employee records should be kept for seven years after the employee leaves and up to 10 years if the employee has filed any kind of work-related accident claim against the business. All ownership records from the business should be kept permanently.

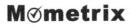

ACCOUNTS RECEIVABLE

Accounts receivable is any money owed to the business owner by an individual or other business owner. A business has accounts receivable when customers are allowed to pay for products or services on credit. Most massage businesses will be a cash business and customers will pay for their service at the time of service. If a customer does not pay at the time of service, an invoice should be created stating the type of service, the amount owed, the date of the service, and the date payment is due. The business owner must be sure to follow up and collect any outstanding accounts receivable debts. If a massage practitioner accepts insurance, there may be outstanding accounts receivables while waiting for the insurance company to pay the claim. The business owner must be sure to manage the accounts receivable so that all expenditures of the business can be paid on time and the business does not have problems paying its own bills.

ACCOUNTS PAYABLE

Accounts payable is the money a business owes to another business or individual. When the business buys materials or supplies on credit, those bills will eventually need to be paid. In an accounting system, accounts payable are considered short-term debt. It is generally outstanding invoices from goods or services purchased by the business that have yet to be paid. For example, if a massage business owner purchases new furniture for the business and receives an invoice to be paid in 30 days, then this would be considered an account payable. It is important to keep a record of these invoices and the disbursements that are paid so that they can be accurately reflected in the profit or loss or income statement. Accounts payable debts that are not paid would be detrimental to the business and to the credit rating of a sole proprietor or business. If accounts payables are not paid on time, other businesses are less likely to allow purchases on credit in the future.

Healthcare and Business Terminology

IMAGINARY PLANES

The three imaginary planes which anatomists use to divide the body are as follows:

- **Sagittal plane** – The sagittal plane divides the body into left and right parts. It is an imaginary line that runs vertically through the body. The term midsagittal is used when the body is being divided into left and right halves.
- **Coronal plane** – The coronal plane is also sometimes referred to as the frontal plane. It divides the body into anterior and posterior, or ventral and dorsal, halves.

Guidelines for Professional Practice

143

- **Transverse plane** – The transverse plane divides the body horizontally into an upper half and a lower half.

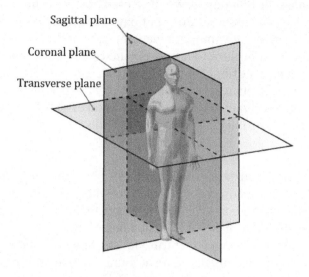

Sagittal plane

Coronal plane

Transverse plane

PROPER ANATOMIC POSITION

Anatomic position is the position in which all directional terms are based on when describing the location of body parts to one another. This position is face forward with arms at sides and palms facing outward.

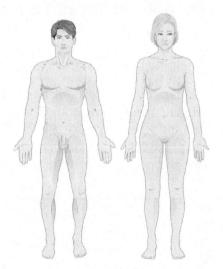

PATHOLOGY

Pathology is the study of disease and the structural and functional changes those diseases cause to the body. It is important for a massage practitioner to understand pathology and how disease affects the body. When disease is present, the body is in an unhealthy and abnormal state. Some diseases can be helped by the aid of massage and others are contraindicated. It is vital that the massage practitioner understand the effects that a specific disease has on the body, the therapeutic effects of massage so that an educated decision can be made as to when to use massage in general, and which specific techniques are appropriate for the client's current condition. For example, massage can be helpful in dealing with the stress and long-term effects of some chronic diseases but

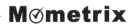

would be contraindicated for many acute illnesses such as the flu or where fever may be present due to massage increasing the core body temperature. A massage practitioner who has a solid understanding of pathology and its effects on the body will better be able to provide proper care for clients.

KINESIOLOGY

Kinesiology is the study of the movement, physiology, anatomy, and mechanics of the human body. A good massage practitioner understands the anatomy of the body and the mechanics of movement. It is vital that a massage practitioner have an understanding of the structures being worked on and how they relate to each other through movement. It is common for a client to feel pain in one area of the body that may actually have a root cause in another part of the body. Understanding this and knowing how to apply the proper massage techniques will allow the massage practitioner to be effective and more likely to assist clients in attaining easier and more pain-free movement. A good massage practitioner must also be able to assess a client. Having a firm grasp of kinesiology will allow the practitioner to make accurate assessments and develop more effective treatment plans. For example, knowing the normal range of motion at the shoulder joint will allow the practitioner to notice restrictions to movement, work to correct them, and provide accurate feedback on the efficacy of the treatment.

FIVE BODY CAVITIES

The body is divided into five body cavities. These cavities are spaces that support, protect, and separate internal organs. The five body cavities are as follows:

- **Cranial cavity** – Formed by the cranial bones. This is where the brain is contained and protected.
- **Spinal cavity** – Formed by the vertebrae. This is where the spinal cord is contained and protected.
- **Thoracic cavity** –Also known as the chest cavity. It is enclosed by ribs, the muscles of the chest, and the thoracic portion of the spinal column. Inside are two smaller cavities that contain the heart and the two lungs.
- **Abdominal cavity** – Located between the diaphragm and the pelvic cavity. It is surrounded by the abdominal wall and contains the stomach, spleen, liver, gallbladder, small intestine, and most of the large intestine.
- **Pelvic cavity** – Located between the bones of the pelvis below the abdominal cavity. It contains the urinary bladder, portions of the large intestine, and internal organs of the reproductive system.

IMPORTANT TERMS

- **Cranial**—Toward the crown of the head.
- **Caudal**—Toward the feet.
- **Anterior**—Located before or in front of.
- **Posterior**—Located behind or in back of.
- **Medial**—Meaning the middle or center, closer to the midline.
- **Lateral**—Meaning on the side, farther away from the midline.
- **Distal**—Pertains to the point the farthest away from the origin of a structure. Relative to the trunk or midline, a distal part would be farther away.
- **Proximal**—Pertains to the point nearest to the origin of a structure or its point of attachment. Relative to the trunk or midline, a proximal part would be nearer.

145

COMMON PREFIXES

Prefix	Definition	Example
Infra	Having a position which is below the part indicated by the word it is attached to.	The *infra*spinatus muscle is beneath the spine of the scapula.
Inter	Refers to being between or among two parts.	The *inter*scapular area is between the two scapulae.
Intra	Meaning occurring or formed within a part.	An *intra*muscular injection is an injection that is given directly into the muscle.
Sub	Meaning less than, beneath, below normal, or typical, inferior.	The *sub*clavian artery is located beneath the clavicle.
Super	Meaning more than normal, excessive, beyond.	There are many new *super*bugs appearing that are resistant to antibiotics.
Supra	Having a position which is above the part indicated by the word it is attached to.	The *supra*spinatus muscle is above the spine of the scapula.

MBLEx Practice Test #1

Want to take this practice test in an online interactive format?
Check out the bonus page, which includes interactive practice questions and much more: **mometrix.com/bonus948/mblex**

SCAN HERE

1. Which of these is an action of the sartorius muscle?

a. Medial rotation of the thigh
b. Extension of the thigh
c. Lateral rotation of the thigh
d. Extension of the knee

2. What is the double-layered membrane that encloses the heart?

a. Bicuspid
b. Pericardium
c. Endocardium
d. Epicardium

3. Which of these conditions would be an absolute contraindication for massage?

a. Fever
b. Edema
c. Pregnancy
d. Diabetes

4. What is the result of respiration?

a. Oxygen and carbon dioxide are exchanged between capillaries and tissue cells.
b. Deoxygenated blood is converted to oxygenated blood.
c. Oxygen diffuses into interstitial fluid then into tissue cells.
d. Carbon dioxide diffuses from tissue cells into the capillaries.

5. Which technique is described as the grasping of the flesh in one or both hands and moving it up and down along the bone?

a. Shaking
b. Chucking
c. Rolling
d. Wringing

6. What is the enlarged area on the end of a long bone that articulates with another bone?

a. Epiphysis
b. Diaphysis
c. Periosteum
d. Articular cartilage

7. Which of these should be included in the preliminary assessment of a new client?

a. Health history
b. Height and weight measurements
c. Resting heart rate
d. Cholesterol check

8. Which of these lower extremity muscles does NOT have an insertion on the femur?

a. Psoas major
b. Tibialis anterior
c. Adductor magnus
d. Gluteus maximus

9. Which of these nerves would be responsible for movement of the eyeball?

a. Trigeminal
b. Olfactory
c. Oculomotor
d. Optic

10. Which of these is a characteristic of diarthrotic joints?

a. Freely moveable
b. Immovable
c. Limited mobility
d. Absence of a joint cavity

11. A client reports during the initial assessment that after shoveling snow at home that morning, there has been a consistent pain on the left side, starting at the jaw and radiating down the left arm. How should the practitioner proceed?

a. Perform range of motion testing on the left side.
b. Spend more time focusing on the left side during the massage.
c. Have the client seek immediate medical attention.
d. Avoid the left side during the massage.

12. Which of these massage techniques is applied in a transverse direction to the tissue being treated?

a. Effleurage
b. Petrissage
c. Cross-fiber friction
d. Chucking

13. What would be the appropriate adjustment to the massage session if a client reports current use of painkillers?

a. Increase the depth of the strokes so that the client can better feel the massage.
b. Decrease the depth of the strokes to prevent tissue damage because sensation may be dulled.
c. No change to the massage session would be necessary.
d. Refuse treatment for this client.

14. Which of these techniques would be used to desensitize a nerve?

a. Wringing
b. Shaking
c. Effleurage
d. Vibration

15. Why must caution be used when treating a client on blood-thinning medication?

a. The client may not be sensitive to pressure.
b. There is increased risk of bruising.
c. There is increased risk of muscle spasm.
d. The client's blood sugar may be high.

16. What is the longest part of the alimentary canal that is lined with small, fingerlike projections called villi?

a. Small intestine
b. Large intestine
c. Digestive tract
d. Esophagus

17. The cubital area of the elbow is an endangerment site. Which of these nerves pass through that area and should be avoided?

a. Sciatic nerve
b. Tibial nerve
c. Optic nerve
d. Median nerve

18. What is the smallest functional unit of a muscle cell?

a. Actin
b. Myosin
c. Sarcomere
d. Spindle

19. Which of these conditions is the accumulation of interstitial fluid in the soft tissue that is caused by blockage, inflammation, or removal of the lymph channels?

a. Hematoma
b. Cancer
c. Lymphedema
d. Phlebitis

20. Which of these conditions involves the inflammation of veins accompanied by pain and swelling?

a. Aneurysm
b. Phlebitis
c. Lymphedema
d. Myocardial infarction

21. What is the effect of light percussion on the blood vessels?

    a. Dilation followed by contraction

    b. Contraction followed by relaxation as movement continues

    c. Continuous contraction until the movement stops

    d. Increased permeability of the vessels

22. Which of these techniques would be applied with the ulnar side of the hand?

    a. Tapping

    b. Jostling

    c. Slapping

    d. Hacking

23. Where are the adrenal glands located?

    a. On the pancreas

    b. On either side of the trachea

    c. On top of each kidney

    d. Behind the thyroid

24. In this type of deep palpation, the tissues are palpated perpendicular to the surface.

    a. Shear

    b. Compression

    c. Superficial

    d. Subcutaneous

25. Which type of muscle contraction results in the distance between the ends of the muscle becoming shorter?

    a. Isotonic contraction

    b. Isometric contraction

    c. Fast-twitch contraction

    d. Slow-twitch contraction

26. When all of the internal systems of the body are in balance, what is this is known as?

    a. Homeopathy

    b. Gate theory

    c. Hyperemia

    d. Homeostasis

27. Which endangerment site is bordered by the sternocleidomastoid and trapezius muscles and the clavicle?

    a. Femoral triangle

    b. Anterior triangle of the neck

    c. Posterior triangle of the neck

    d. Popliteal fossa

28. Which of these is NOT a factor in determining scope of practice?

    a. Activities that are legally acceptable according to the licenses of the profession

    b. The age and sex of the practitioner

    c. Training received by the practitioner

    d. Choice of preferred clientele

29. Which of these would NOT be a benefit of massage to the critically ill?

    a. Decreases pain receptors
    b. Reduces disorientation
    c. Reduces isolation
    d. Improves mobility

30. Which of these massage techniques would be stimulating to the nervous system?

    a. Gentle stroking
    b. Light friction
    c. Vibration
    d. Ischemic compression

31. What is the benefit of ischemic compression?

    a. Increases adrenaline
    b. Stimulates the peripheral nerves
    c. Releases the reflex cycle that maintains hypertension in the muscle
    d. Increases lymph flow to the extremities

32. Which of the following would be considered an open-ended question?

    a. Do you smoke?
    b. Do you have a referral from a physician?
    c. How would you describe your current pain level?
    d. Have you had a surgery in the past?

33. Which of these is NOT a principal function of the skin?

    a. Protection
    b. Heat regulation
    c. Absorption
    d. Regrowth

34. A vertical plumb line running from above the head along the lateral side of the body to the floor, when viewed from the side, would pass through which of these structures?

    a. Pubic symphysis
    b. Iliac crest
    c. Acromioclavicular joint
    d. Acetabulum

35. Which of these muscles has an attachment site on the clavicle?

    a. Levator scapulae
    b. Pectoralis major
    c. Pectoralis minor
    d. Teres major

36. During a visual assessment, the practitioner observes that the client's right shoulder is elevated. Which of the following muscles is most likely involved?

    a. Levator scapulae
    b. Pectoralis minor
    c. Lower trapezius
    d. Rhomboid major

37. What is an acute inflammation caused by the herpes zoster virus that creates inflammation at a nerve trunk and the dendrites at the end of the sensory neurons called?

    a. Neuritis
    b. Polio
    c. Meningitis
    d. Shingles

38. While palpating the neck the practitioner may feel these small nodules, which are between the size of a pea and a kidney bean.

    a. Pineal glands
    b. Ganglia
    c. Lymph nodes
    d. Facet joints

39. Which of these is an effect of increased serotonin levels?

    a. An increase in feelings of stress
    b. An increase in food cravings
    c. A higher incidence of eating disorders
    d. An increase in feelings of calm and well-being

40. What is the bony prominence that can be palpated at the hip joint?

    a. Greater tubercle
    b. Greater trochanter
    c. Acromion
    d. Femoral tuberosity

41. Which of these would be considered a form of nonverbal communication?

    a. Sighing
    b. Frowning
    c. Whispering
    d. Questioning

42. Which of these types of barriers is the first sign of resistance to a movement?

    a. Anatomic barrier
    b. Physiologic barrier
    c. End barrier
    d. Resistive barrier

43. A client is two months post-surgery and cleared for massage. Which of these techniques would be most effective for aligning the scar tissue at the surgical site?

    a. Tapping
    b. Cross-fiber friction
    c. Petrissage
    d. Vibration

44. What is the largest lymph vessel of the body?

a. Cervical lymph nodes
b. Thoracic duct
c. Spleen
d. Internal jugular

45. What is a form of energetic manipulation often used in hospitals by nurses?

a. Neuromuscular therapy
b. Myofascial release
c. Therapeutic touch
d. Alexander technique

46. What is the purpose of Golgi tendon organs?

a. To sense the movement and position of joints
b. To activate muscle contraction
c. To maintain balance
d. To measure the amount of tension in a muscle due to stretching and contracting

47. What is a set of guiding moral principles that directs a person's choice of actions and behaviors?

a. Professional boundary
b. Therapeutic relationship
c. Code of ethics
d. Ethical arrangement

48. Why is massage in the supine position for more than ten to fifteen minutes not recommended after the twentieth week of pregnancy?

a. The uterus can put pressure on the major lymph and blood vessels of the abdomen.
b. The ligaments and joints are too loose to maintain the position.
c. There will be too much pressure on the lungs.
d. It tends to make the fetus very active.

49. Which of these would NOT be a way for a practitioner to maintain appropriate interpersonal space with a client before and after the massage?

a. Carry on conversations at eye level.
b. Remain standing while the client is seated.
c. Complete most of the important conversation before the client is on the table.
d. Maintain a comfortable distance from the client while talking.

50. Which of these hormones causes acceleration in heart rate and inhibition of the digestive system?

a. Epinephrine
b. Dopamine
c. Estrogen
d. Melatonin

MBLEx Practice Test #1

51. A client comments during the massage that a coworker is also receiving massage from the practitioner and enquires about the coworker's condition. How should the practitioner respond?

a. The practitioner should inform the client that it is against confidentiality guidelines to share personal information.
b. The practitioner should give a brief summary of the client's condition without divulging too much information.
c. The practitioner should encourage the client to talk to his or her coworker about the condition.
d. The practitioner should ask the client if the coworker has reported satisfactory progress from the massage.

52. What is it called when a client gives written authorization for professional services based on the client's full understanding of the expectations, benefits, and any undesirable effects?

a. A treatment plan
b. Explanation of benefits
c. Informed consent
d. Consultation

53. Which of these would be a code of ethics violation according to the National Certification Board for Therapeutic Massage and Bodywork's Code of Ethics?

a. Refuse to treat a client because the practitioner does not feel competent to treat the client's condition.
b. Provide treatment only when there is a reasonable expectation that it would be advantageous to the client.
c. Attend continuing education.
d. Accept gifts from a client who has had extraordinary results from treatment.

54. A client complains of lower back pain during the massage. Where is this information documented on a SOAP chart?

a. Objective
b. Subjective
c. Assessment or applications
d. Planning

55. A client invites the practitioner out for drinks with friends after the massage. How should the practitioner respond?

a. The practitioner should ask where and what time.
b. The practitioner should suggest a meal before drinks.
c. The practitioner should tell the client that drinking after massage is not recommended.
d. The practitioner should gently inform the client that personal relationships outside of the massage setting are not appropriate.

56. What is a Japanese finger pressure technique that affects the circulation of fluids and chi?

a. Reiki
b. Shiatsu
c. Ayurveda
d. Anatripsis

57. Slow, rhythmic massage of which of these areas can elicit a sexual response?

    a. Lower back
    b. Feet
    c. Lower abdomen
    d. Hands

58. What is the definition of the word *anatripsis*?

    a. Rubbing of the head to relieve headache
    b. The lifting and grasping of the tissues to make space between the tissues
    c. The art of rubbing a part upward, not downward
    d. The rubbing of the limbs to strengthen the muscles and combat paralysis

59. Which form should be signed by the client to provide an update of status to the client's physician?

    a. Health history form
    b. Release of information form
    c. HIPAA form
    d. SOAP chart

60. Which of these is a stance where the practitioner stands with both feet in line with the edge of the table and moves by shifting the weight side to side?

    a. Archer stance
    b. Horse stance
    c. Saddle stance
    d. Grounding stance

61. Which of these is NOT a characteristic of licensing?

    a. Is issued by a governmental agency
    b. Is voluntary to show proficiency or accomplishment
    c. Specifies a scope of practice
    d. Determines minimum requirements for compliance

62. Which of these types of muscles is involuntary, nonstriated, and can maintain a contraction for a long period of time?

    a. Smooth muscle
    b. Cardiac muscle
    c. Skeletal muscle
    d. Fast twitch muscle

63. Which of these would be a reason for a license to be revoked, suspended, or canceled?

    a. Accepting a large tip from a client
    b. Asking a client about his or her divorce
    c. Prescribing drugs
    d. Practicing new massage techniques on a client

MBLEx Practice Test #1

64. Which of these would be classified as a synarthrotic joint?

a. Sutures of the skull
b. Sacroiliac joint
c. Hip joint
d. Shoulder joint

65. What are personal comfort zones that help a person maintain a feeling of comfort and safety?

a. Boundaries
b. Ethics
c. Morals
d. Values

66. What accommodations should a massage practitioner make when working with a frail, elderly client?

a. No accommodations need to be made as long as the client is healthy.
b. Require the client to have a friend or family member assist them onto the table.
c. Use a lighter touch because the tissues are more delicate and susceptible to bruising.
d. Frail, elderly clients should not receive massage.

67. How can a practitioner set boundaries related to time?

a. Always finish the massage early so the next appointment can start on time.
b. Set policies regarding no shows and late arrivals.
c. Tell clients that the appointment time is fifteen minutes before the scheduled time to ensure early arrival.
d. Don't schedule appointments after 7:00 pm.

68. According to this theory, stimulation of thermo- or mechanoreceptors using massage, ice, or rubbing will suppress pain sensations where the fibers enter the spinal column.

a. Pain control theory
b. Mechanical control theory
c. Gate control theory
d. Sensory control theory

69. What is the ideal temperature range for the massage room?

a. 68 to 72 degrees Fahrenheit
b. 72 to 75 degrees Fahrenheit
c. 76 to 80 degrees Fahrenheit
d. 62 to 66 degrees Fahrenheit

70. Which of these is NOT a goal of the initial consultation?

a. Establish open communication with the client
b. Perform a preliminary assessment
c. Obtain informed consent
d. Palpate for muscular imbalances

71. The practitioner begins to cough excessively during the massage. What is the appropriate course of action?

  a. Cough in to the sleeve and continue the massage.
  b. Apologize for being so loud.
  c. Apologize and leave the room to get water and wash hands thoroughly before returning.
  d. Offer the client a discount.

72. In which section of a SOAP chart should the results of range of motion testing be recorded?

  a. Objective
  b. Subjective
  c. Assessment or applications
  d. Planning

73. What is the system of infection control created to protect persons from blood and blood borne pathogens?

  a. Universal precautions
  b. Sterilization
  c. Disinfecting
  d. Safety protocol

74. Who made gymnastics and the regular use of massage part of their physical fitness rituals?

  a. Greeks
  b. Japanese
  c. Chinese
  d. Hindu

75. What is the proper bleach-to-water solution ratio for disinfecting surfaces?

  a. 1:5
  b. 1:100
  c. 1:20
  d. 1:10

76. Which of these is NOT an endangerment site?

  a. Medial brachium
  b. Popliteal fossa
  c. Upper lumbar area
  d. Quadriceps triangle

77. Which of the following would be a reason for the practitioner to wear vinyl gloves during the massage?

  a. When the client has soiled feet
  b. When the practitioner has sweaty hands
  c. When the practitioner has an open wound on the hand
  d. When the client has a fever

78. What is the term for when a practitioner develops strong emotional feelings toward a client?

   a. Countertransference
   b. Transference
   c. Dual relationship
   d. Abusive

79. How can a practitioner use leverage to apply deeper pressure without using muscle strength from the hands and arms?

   a. Climb onto the table.
   b. Use the elbows.
   c. Stand on the toes.
   d. Lean into the technique.

80. What are the rights and activities that are legally acceptable under the license of a particular profession defined by?

   a. Code of ethics
   b. Certification
   c. Local ordinance
   d. Scope of practice

81. Where is the proper position for a bolster when the client is lying on the table in the supine position?

   a. Behind the knees
   b. Under the ankles
   c. Under the lower back
   d. None at all

82. Which of these types of neurons carries a signal indicating pain from a sense organ to the brain?

   a. Efferent neurons
   b. Interneurons
   c. Neurotransmitter
   d. Afferent neurons

83. How can a practitioner secure the draping while the client is rolling over?

   a. Lift the sheet off of the table.
   b. Ask the client to hold onto the drape while rolling over.
   c. Use an extra-long sheet on top.
   d. Lean on the table.

84. Which of the following would NOT be an inert tissue?

   a. Bursa
   b. Nerve
   c. Ligament
   d. Tendon

85. What is a short, general statement that defines the main focus of a business?

a. Mission statement
b. Business plan
c. Purpose
d. Strategic plan

86. A new client reports during the initial interview that there has been a recent diagnosis of cancer and treatments have not yet begun. How should the massage practitioner continue?

a. The practitioner should request a doctor's recommendation before treating the client.
b. The practitioner should perform a full-body massage and avoid the area of the body that is affected by the cancer.
c. The practitioner should call the treating physician's office and ask for permission to treat the client.
d. The practitioner should refer the client to another massage practitioner who has experience treating cancer patients.

87. Which of these would be a characteristic of being an independent contractor, according to the Internal Revenue Service?

a. Receiving vacation days
b. Hours of work set by the business owner
c. Freedom to set own hours
d. Taxes withheld from the paycheck

88. Which of these would NOT be a benefit of massage to a person with cancer?

a. Increases blood flow to tumor site
b. Boosts the healing process
c. Reduces edema
d. Improves flow of lymph

89. What is a business setup that is subject to regulation and taxation and requires a charter?

a. Sole proprietorship
b. Corporation
c. Partnership
d. Limited liability company

90. Which of the following is NOT an inert tissue?

a. Tendon
b. Ligament
c. Bursa
d. Nerve

91. Which organ of the digestive system contains glands that produce hydrochloric acid?

a. Gallbladder
b. Stomach
c. Pancreas
d. Large Intestine

92. Which of these advanced massage modalities most addresses trigger points and their relationship to local and referred pain?
   a.   Myofascial release
   b.   Therapeutic touch
   c.   Muscle energy technique
   d.   Neuromuscular therapy

93. What is the origin of the anterior fibers of the deltoid muscle?
   a.   Lateral one-third of the clavicle
   b.   Lesser tubercle of the humerus
   c.   Costal cartilage of ribs one through six
   d.   Deltoid tuberosity of the humerus

94. Which plexus of the nervous system supplies the abdominal organs?
   a.   Brachial plexus
   b.   Cervical plexus
   c.   Lumbar plexus
   d.   Sacral plexus

95. Which of these is an example of a dual relationship?
   a.   When a client is referred to the massage practitioner by a physician
   b.   When the practitioner refers the client to another massage practitioner
   c.   When the client is requesting massage for more than one condition
   d.   When the client and practitioner belong to the same social organization

96. What is the muscle that performs the opposite movement of the prime mover?
   a.   Fixator
   b.   Agonist
   c.   Antagonist
   d.   Synergist

97. What are the three types of end feels that are considered normal?
   a.   Hard, soft, springy
   b.   Springy, empty, hard
   c.   Soft, empty, short
   d.   Hard, inert, springy

98. Which of the following drugs is classified as a non-opioid analgesic?
   a.   Percocet
   b.   Morphine
   c.   Demerol
   d.   Tylenol

99. What is the term for when a client attempts to personalize the relationship with the massage practitioner by projecting characteristics of someone from a previous relationship?
   a.   Countertransference
   b.   Duality
   c.   Transference
   d.   Therapeutic

100. A client is being seen for muscular tightness in the low back that has been evaluated by a physician. The physician referred the client for massage after finding no injury. The client reports that after six massage sessions, there has been no change in symptoms. How should the practitioner proceed?

    a. The practitioner should reassess the client to evaluate whether a change in treatment is justified.

    b. The practitioner should proceed with the massage as stated in the treatment plan.

    c. The practitioner should refuse treatment to the client.

    d. The practitioner should refer the client to another physician.

Answer Key and Explanations for Test #1

1. C: The sartorius muscle has multiple actions. It flexes, laterally rotates, abducts the thigh, and assists with flexion and medial rotation of the knee.

2. B: The pericardium is the double-layered membrane that encloses the heart. It is made up of two layers, a thin inner layer, which provides a serous covering for the heart, and an outer layer made up of fibrous connective tissue, which serves as protection.

3. A: Massage is contraindicated when fever is present. Normal body temperature is 98.6 degrees Fahrenheit. If the client feels abnormally warm, the temperature should be taken. Most physicians and therapists will advise against massage when the body temperature is above 99.4 degrees Fahrenheit. Fever is the body's natural defense system against an invading pathogen. Massage could disrupt this natural process.

4. B: External respiration happens in the lungs. It is when deoxygenated blood that is coming from the right side of the heart is oxygenated and returned to the left side of the heart. It is an exchange of oxygen and carbon dioxide between the air in the alveoli of the lungs and the blood of the pulmonary capillaries.

5. B: Chucking is a technique that is described as the grasping of flesh in one or both hands and moving it up and down along the bone. It is performed as a series of quick movements along the axis of the bone. It is considered a friction movement.

6. A: A long bone has an enlarged area on each end, the epiphysis, which serves as an articulation point for other bones. The epiphysis is covered with a layer of hyaline cartilage known as the articular cartilage. This provides a smooth surface for the two bones to form a joint. The articular cartilage also provides a shock-absorbing surface for the articulation.

7. A: In the preliminary assessment the massage practitioner needs to understand as much about the client as possible. Depending on the type of massage being offered, the assessment may be more superficial or more in depth. The practitioner should always be sure to take a thorough health history of the client to be aware of any contraindications or cautions to make an informed decision regarding the treatment plan.

8. B: The tibialis anterior does not have an attachment on the femur. This muscle originates at the lateral and proximal one half of the tibia and the interosseous membrane and inserts in to the medial and plantar surface of the medial cuneiform and the base of the first metatarsal.

9. C: The oculomotor nerve is the third cranial nerve. It controls the movement of the eyelid and the eyeball and causes constriction of the pupil. It originates in the midbrain and passes through the superior orbital fissure. It is considered primarily a motor nerve.

10. A: Diarthrotic joints are freely moveable joints. These joints have an articular cartilage and are surrounded by a joint capsule that contains synovial fluid that lubricates the joint surfaces. They are capable of different kinds of movements. Some examples of diarthrotic joints are pivot joints, hinge joints, ball and socket joints, and saddle joints.

11. C: If a client reports pain in the left arm, this can be a sign of a heart attack. Pain radiating down from the jaw on to the left side is often an early sign of heart attack. Shoveling snow is a very common cause of heart attack, especially in those who are sedentary. Someone demonstrating

162

these symptoms should seek medical attention immediately to rule out a heart-related condition. Other signs of heart attack would be shortness of breath, lightheadedness, and chest pain.

12. C: Cross-fiber friction is applied in a transverse direction with the tips of the fingers or the thumb. It is applied across the fibers of muscle, tendon, or ligament with the intent to break up adhesions and scar tissue, align the fibers, and broaden and separate the tissue.

13. B: If a client reports current use of painkillers, the practitioner should decrease the depth of the strokes to prevent tissue damage because sensation may be dulled and tissue response may not be normal. The client may not be able to accurately report the proper pressure tolerance after taking painkillers. It is recommended that the client receive massage at the end of the dosage regimen so that pain information is more accurate.

14. D: Vibration is a technique that can be done manually or with an electronic device. When vibrations are applied for a prolonged period it has an anesthetizing effect. It is often used to desensitize nerves or areas of the body.

15. B: Blood thinners or anticoagulants such as Heparin and Warfarin are used to prevent blood from clotting. Caution must be used on clients who are taking blood thinners. The risk of bruising or internal bleeding is increased, especially in the elderly.

16. A: The small intestine is part of the digestive system and is the longest part of the alimentary canal. The small intestine contains three parts: the duodenum, jejunum, and ileum. Villi are the small, fingerlike projections that increase the surface area of the small intestine and allow for greater absorption.

17. D: The cubital area is the anterior bend of the elbow. It is an endangerment site because the median nerve, radial and ulnar arteries, and median cubital vein pass through this area. These can be easily compressed if deep manipulations or direct sustained pressure occurs at this site.

18. C: The smallest functional unit of a muscle cell is the sarcomere. Inside each sarcomere are the proteins myosin and actin. The myosin and actin line up to create the striated appearance of skeletal muscle. The activity of the actin and myosin filaments in the sarcomere is what gives muscle its contractile ability.

19. C: Lymphedema is a swelling that occurs when interstitial fluid accumulates in the soft tissue, usually in the extremities. The fluid is unable to pass due a blockage, inflammation, or removal of lymph channels. It can be caused by surgery, trauma, radiation, or infection. It can also occur due to a congenital or genetic condition that prevents the lymph system from developing completely.

20. B: Phlebitis is the inflammation of veins that is accompanied by pain and swelling. It can be caused by infection, injury, or surgery or have no known cause. A blood clot can form along the inflamed vein and develop into a condition known as deep vein thrombosis (DVT).

21. B: Light percussion strokes will initially cause the blood vessels to contract, but with continued movement there will be a relaxation of the blood vessels.

22. D: Hacking is a rapid striking movement that is done with the little finger and the ulnar side of the hand. It can be performed with one or both hands. The wrist and fingers should remain loose and relaxed with the fingers spread apart slightly. The fingers will come together as the hand strikes the body, causing a vibratory effect.

23. C: The adrenal glands are located on the top of each kidney and are made of up two parts, the medulla and the adrenal cortex. The medulla produces epinephrine and norepinephrine. The adrenal cortex produces corticosteroids.

24. B: Compression is a form of deep palpation. The tissue is palpated through layers perpendicular to the surface. Compression is often used to palpate muscle and its associated structures.

25. A: A muscle contraction that results in the distance between the ends of the muscle becoming shorter is an isotonic contraction. When the distance between the ends of the muscle becomes shorter, this is known as a concentric isotonic contraction. The opposite contraction, when the distance between the ends of the muscle becomes longer, is known as an eccentric isotonic contraction. All isotonic contractions cause changes in the distance between the ends of a muscle.

26. D: Homeostasis is the body's natural internal balance. It is maintained by the work of both the sympathetic and parasympathetic nervous systems. The body strives to remain in a state of homeostasis.

27. C: The posterior triangle of the neck is an endangerment site on the body that is bordered by the sternocleidomastoid muscle, the trapezius muscle, and the clavicle. It contains the brachial plexus, the subclavian artery, the external jugular vein, and lymph nodes. All of these are structures of concern, and caution must be used when massaging in this area.

28. B: The scope of practice is determined by what is legally acceptable under the license of the practitioner. Factors that also influence a practitioner's scope of practice are the skills and interests of the practitioner, the training received, and the type of clientele the practitioner would like to work with.

29. A: Massage has no effect on the number of pain receptors in the body. It can help those who are critically ill by reducing disorientation and isolation and improving mobility. Massage also helps with discomfort and pain and eases emotional strain.

30. C: Vibration movements such as shaking and trembling will stimulate the peripheral nerves and all nerve centers associated with a specific nerve trunk.

31. C: Ischemic compression or, holding of pressure, on a sensitive trigger point can release the reflex cycle that is maintaining hypertension in a muscle. It does this by desensitizing the trigger point, which stops the pathophysiological reflex cycle from continuing.

32. C: When questioning a client regarding current concerns and any health issues that are present, the practitioner should ask open-ended questions. Open-ended questions are ones that cannot be answered with a simple yes or no and require further explanation. This allows the practitioner to better understand the client's needs and health situation.

33. D: The principal functions of the skin are: protection, heat regulation, secretion and excretion, sensation, absorption, and respiration.

34. D: A vertical plumb line that runs from the head to the floor when viewed from the side should pass through the ear, shoulder, elbow, acetabulum, knee, and just in front of the ankle. This plumb line can be used to detect postural deviations or abnormalities in clients as part of the assessment process.

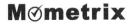

35. B: The pectoralis major has two heads, the clavicular and sternal. The clavicular head originates at the clavicle and inserts into the lateral ridge of the bicipital groove of the humerus. The sternal head originates at the sternum and costal cartilages of ribs one through six and inserts into the lateral ridge of the bicipital groove of the humerus.

36. A: The levator scapulae muscle originates on the transverse processes of C1–C4 and inserts into the superior one-third of the vertebral border of the scapula. The actions of the levator scapulae are elevation of the scapula and lateral flexion of the neck. If this muscle is hypertonic, it can hold the scapula in an elevated position and would be visible upon observation.

37. D: Shingles is an acute inflammation caused by the herpes zoster virus. It causes inflammation of a nerve trunk and the dendrites at the end of sensory neurons. Shingles presents as a rash with water blisters that appears in a confined area on one side of the body. The rash will seldom cross the midline. The virus causes a band of pain that follows the dermatomes of the body. Massage is contraindicated due to pain and risk of infection.

38. C: Lymph nodes can be palpated on the sides of the neck, in the axillary region, or in the inguinal area. They are small nodules between the size of a pea and a kidney bean. At times they can be enlarged due to illness. If a practitioner palpates enlarged lymph nodes, it should be brought to the attention of the client.

39. D: Serotonin is a neurotransmitter. It has many influences on the body including affecting mood, behavior, appetite, blood pressure, temperature regulation, memory, and learning ability. It counters the effects of norepinephrine, promotes a sense of calm and well-being, suppresses irritability, and reduces cravings for food and sex.

40. B: The greater trochanter is the bony knob at the top of the femur. It can be easily palpated at the hip. It is an attachment site for many muscles, including the gluteus maximus and the lateral rotators of the hip.

41. B: Frowning is a form of nonverbal communication. Nonverbal communication is posturing, gestures, and facial expressions that express a person's mental, emotional, or physical state. It is important for a massage practitioner to observe these nonverbal clues as well as verbal feedback from the client.

42. D: The first sign of resistance to a movement is the resistive barrier. It is well within the anatomical limits of the involved tissues. It is the bind felt when the contractile tissue is reaching the outer limits of its range of motion. Incremental force can be used to move past this barrier and on to the physiologic and anatomic barriers.

43. B: Cross-fiber friction is applied using the tips of the fingers or the thumb directly to the site of a lesion or scar. It is applied in a transverse direction to the fibers. The intent of cross-fiber friction is to align fibrous tissue, break up adhesions, and soften scar tissue.

44. B: The thoracic duct, also known as the left lymphatic duct, is the largest lymphatic vessel of the body. It collects lymph from the legs, abdomen, left arm, and left side of the head, neck, and chest. The lymph from the thoracic duct reenters the bloodstream at the left subclavian vein and from there flows to the heart.

45. C: Therapeutic touch is a simple form of bodywork that is very popular with nurses. It is based on the belief that all people have the inherent ability to heal and that anyone can be a vessel for

Answer Key and Explanations for Test #1

165

healing. The purpose is to balance the energy fields and aura of the body by contacting them with the hands held above and off of the body.

46. D: Golgi tendon organs can be found at the musculotendinous junction, where tendons attach to muscle fibers. They are sensory nerve organs that sense the amount of tension in the muscle cells due to the stretching and contracting of the muscle. They also measure the amount of force on the bone at the tendon attachment.

47. C: A profession is generally represented by a professional association regulated and guided by a code of ethics. A code of ethics is a set of moral principles that direct the professional's choice of actions. Both the National Certification Board for Therapeutic Massage and Bodywork and the American Massage Therapy Association have codes of ethics that guide massage practitioners toward making ethical and professional choices.

48. A: After the twentieth week of pregnancy, massage longer than ten to fifteen minutes should be avoided in the supine position due to the increasing size of the uterus, which can put pressure on the major lymph and blood vessels of the abdomen. Safer positioning, such as a semi-reclining position, which places the torso at an elevated forty-five- to seventy-degree angle is recommended. A small bolster could be placed under the right shoulder and hip during supine massage to give a left lateral tilt to the uterus, which will prevent it from placing pressure on the abdominal vena cava and aorta.

49. B: Interpersonal space is the physical space maintained between the client and practitioner before and after the massage. This space should make both parties comfortable. It is important to respect the height and power differential while maintaining personal space. It is best that conversations are held at eye level whenever possible. Both parties should either sit or stand while speaking. When one party is much taller of if one party is seated while the other party stands, this gives a sense of power to the person at a greater height.

50. A: Epinephrine is the body's fight-or-flight hormone. Epinephrine is secreted by the adrenal glands to prepare the body to respond to stress or emergencies. It accelerates the heart rate and activates sweat glands. The blood flow is diverted away from digestion and toward the muscles, which inhibits digestion and prepares the body for activity.

51. A: Maintaining client confidentiality is extremely important. The practitioner must never divulge information about another client without that client's permission in writing. Any time that an enquiry is made about another client, no matter the relationship, the practitioner must inform that person that it is against confidentiality guidelines to share personal information about a current or former client.

52. C: Informed consent is the process of the practitioner providing enough information to the client so that the client is able to fully understand the nature and extent of the massage services being offered. The client is given disclosure of the services, policies, and procedures as well as information on benefits and side effects. With this information, the client is able to give informed consent to proceed with treatment. It is recommended that the client sign an informed consent form before receiving massage.

53. D: According to the code of ethics of the National Certification Board for Therapeutic Massage and Bodywork, a massage practitioner should "refuse any gifts or benefits that are intended to influence a referral, decision, or treatment or that are purely for personal gain and not for the good of the client." A client may show appreciation by giving a tip to the practitioner, as is customary, but gifts should not be accepted.

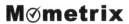

54. B: The subjective, or S, section of a SOAP chart is where the client's reporting of symptoms, aggravating or relieving activities, and pain levels are documented. This is not measurable or observable data but the subjective reporting of the client. Also included in this section would be the client's experiences, expectations, and goals.

55. D: If a client asks the practitioner to participate in social activities outside of the massage setting, the practitioner should gently turn down the request. It is important to maintain professional and personal boundaries with a client. Socializing with a client could lead to more serious ethical violations and disrupt the therapeutic relationship.

56. B: The Japanese massage technique known as Shiatsu is used to affect the circulation of fluids and chi. Finger pressure is used to stimulate nerves that are aligned to the Chinese pressure points used in acupressure. These points are believed to increase the flow of fluids and the life force, known as chi, throughout the body.

57. C: Any time that a practitioner provides slow, rhythmic massage in the lower abdomen area, as well as the buttocks and thighs, it is possible to elicit a sexual response in the client. A sexual response can be easily recognized as a penile erection in males. In women it is not as obvious but can be demonstrated by flushing of the skin and fidgeting.

58. C: Anatripsis is the rubbing of a part upward, not downward. This word was used by Hippocrates in his writings on massage.

59. B: Under HIPAA laws created in 2001, a health practitioner who stores or transmits personal health information electronically must not divulge any client information to a third party without first obtaining a written release of information form that is signed by the client. Massage practitioners may not be required to be HIPAA compliant but should always strive to maintain the highest level of confidentiality for clients.

60. B: The horse stance is used most often when kneading the back and the legs. The practitioner's feet are in line with the edge of the table, and movement is applied by shifting the weight from side to side. The practitioner can lean into the client for deeper pressure. In this posture the back should be relaxed and erect with the shoulders dropped down and back.

61. B: Licensing is a requirement for conducting a business or practicing a particular trade or craft. A license is issued by a regulating agency of the state or municipality. It sets the minimum requirements for compliance in that profession, specifies a scope of practice, and must be renewed at predetermined intervals.

62. A: Smooth muscle is involuntary and controlled by the autonomic nervous system. The cells are nonstriated and spindle shaped and will commonly form fibrous bands. Smooth muscle is found in the stomach, intestines, and blood vessels. It does not attach to bone, can hold a contraction for a long time, and will not easily fatigue.

63. C: Prescribing drugs would be a reason for a license to be revoked, suspended, or canceled. Other reasons for license suspension, cancellation, or revocation would be fraud in obtaining the license, being convicted of a felony, acts of prostitution, practicing under a false or assumed name, being addicted to narcotics or alcohol, being negligent in the practice of massage, ethical or sexual misconduct, and practicing beyond the scope permitted by law.

64. A: The sutures of the skull are classified as synarthrotic joints. A synarthrotic joint is one that is classified as essentially immovable. This is the functional classification of a joint. Joints can also be classified according to their structure.

65. A: Boundaries are a way for a person to maintain a feeling of comfort and safety. They are personal comfort zones that can be professional, personal, physical, emotional, intellectual, or sexual. To have a healthy therapeutic relationship with a client, a practitioner must understand and respect personal and professional boundaries.

66. C: The tissue of the frail elderly is delicate and more susceptible to bruising. Care must be taken when massaging elderly or frail clients. Many times, the skin is paper thin and is easily damaged. A lighter touch is recommended.

67. B: It is important for a massage practitioner to set clear professional boundaries related to time. The practitioner should set clear policies regarding no shows and late arrivals so that the client understands the boundaries and knows what to expect regarding scheduling and arriving on time for the massage.

68. C: Gate control theory states that impulses of pain are transmitted from the nociceptors to the brain via both small- and large-diameter nerve fibers. Stimulation of thermo- or mechanoreceptors is transmitted via large-diameter fibers only. When thermo- or mechanoreceptors are stimulated through massage, ice, or rubbing, those sensations suppress the pain sensations at the gate where the fibers enter the spinal column, thus blocking those sensations from being sent to the brain.

69. B: The ideal temperature for a massage room is 72 to 75 degrees Fahrenheit. This temperature will prevent the client from becoming too cold while on the table and also prevent the practitioner from becoming too warm while performing the massage.

70. D: During the initial consultation with a client, the goals of the practitioner should include establishing a rapport with the client, explaining policies and procedures, determining the needs and expectations of the client, reviewing the health history and intake forms, performing a preliminary assessment, formulating a treatment plan, and obtaining informed consent. Palpation for muscular imbalances would be a part of the ongoing assessment process that happens during the massage.

71. C: If the massage practitioner begins to cough excessively during the massage, the practitioner should apologize to the client for the disruption and leave the room to get water to quiet the cough. Once the coughing has subsided, the practitioner should wash hands thoroughly and return to the room.

72. A: In the objective, or O, section of a SOAP chart, the practitioner reports information that is gathered from observation, interviewing, and assessment tests. This information should be measurable data or the observations of the practitioner. The practitioner's treatment goals should also be included in this section.

73. A: Universal precautions are a system of infection control created to protect persons from blood and blood-borne pathogens. It assumes that all blood and bodily fluids are potentially infectious from diseases such as HIV and hepatitis. It lays out the specific procedures for handling bodily fluids and cleaning linens and surfaces that have come in contact with blood and other bodily fluids.

74. A: The Greeks were the first to combine the modalities of exercise and massage and were the founders of the first gymnasium. Gymnasiums were where physical fitness rituals using massage

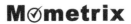

and exercise were performed. The gymnasiums were an important part of Greek life and served as centers where scholars, athletes, soldiers, and the sick came to be treated for disease and to promote health.

75. D: Chlorine bleach is an effective disinfectant for surfaces, implements, and linens. For surfaces and implements, a 1:10 solution should be prepared. Combine one-part bleach to nine parts water. Implements should be immersed in the solution for ten minutes. For linens one cup bleach can be added to hot water during the wash cycle.

76. D: The medial brachium, popliteal fossa, and upper lumbar are all endangerment sites on the body. These areas all have major nerves, blood vessels, or vital organs that are exposed. Deep manipulation or direct, sustained pressure should be avoided in these areas.

77. C: A practitioner should wear vinyl gloves or another appropriate type of coverage anytime there is broken skin or any type of infection on the hands. This is to protect both the client and practitioner.

78. A: When a practitioner begins to personalize the therapeutic relationship with a client, this is known as countertransference. Signs of countertransference are strong emotional feelings toward the client, thinking excessively about a client between sessions, wearing special clothing when a certain client is coming, spending extra time with a client, having sexual feelings about a client, having feelings of dread about upcoming appointments with a certain client, or having negative reactions to a client.

79. D: To apply deeper pressure without using muscle strength from the hands and arms, a massage practitioner can use leverage by leaning into the technique. The practitioner, as a general rule, should stay behind the area being worked on instead of in front of it. This will allow for better leverage and body alignment.

80. D: Scope of practice is the set of rights and activities that have been defined as legally acceptable according to the licenses of a particular profession. This definition should be described in the licensing regulation. The education process of the profession helps determine the scope of practice. The skills learned and training received is directly related to the scope of practice of the occupation.

81. A: When the client is lying in the supine position, a bolster should be used behind the knees to reduce tension in the low back and back of the legs.

82. D: Afferent neurons carry signals of touch, cold, heat, sight, hearing, taste, or pain from the sensory organs of the body to the brain, where they are interpreted.

83. D: When the client is rolling over, the practitioner can secure the draping by leaning into the table and holding the drape in place while grasping the drape at the level of the client's shoulders and hips. The drape can then be lifted to allow the client to reposition and remain secure.

84. D: A tendon is not inert tissue. It is contractile tissue. Muscle and tendon are contractile tissues. Inert tissues are not contractile.

85. A: A mission statement expresses the values of the business. It is a short, general statement that explains the main focus of the business. It can be used in advertising and promotional materials and should be carefully considered. This is the statement that reflects the business's public image.

Answer Key and Explanations for Test #1

86. A: The practitioner should always request a doctor's recommendation before treating a client with cancer. It is important to work closely with the client's medical team and have a full understanding of the illness and current treatment plan. The practitioner should remain in contact with the physician to be aware of any change in condition and treatment recommendations.

87. C: There are three criteria the Internal Revenue Service uses to define a relationship as an independent contractor as opposed to an employee. One criterion is that the independent contractor must be able to set the work hours and the manner in which the work is done. An independent contractor must also have financial control by paying either a flat fee or rent or receiving commission based on work completed. The independent contractor does not receive vacation pay, sick days, or benefits. The independent contractor relationship is usually defined in a contract signed by both parties.

88. A: Increasing blood flow to the tumor site is not a benefit of massage to a person with cancer. Massage will boost the healing process, reduce edema, and improve lymph flow. It will also relieve stress, promote relaxation, help with insomnia, and reduce anxiety as well as many other benefits.

89. B: A corporation is a legal business entity that is separate from any individual or individuals. A charter must be obtained in the state the corporation is operating in. The corporation is managed by a board of directors and has stockholders who share in the profits but are not legally responsible for the actions of the corporation. The corporation is taxed separately from any shareholders.

90. A: Inert tissue is any tissue that is not contractile. This would include bone, ligament, bursa, nerve, blood vessels, and cartilage. Tendon and muscle are contractile tissues.

91. B: Food passes through the esophagus and in to the stomach. Gastric juices containing hydrochloric acid and digestive enzymes mix with the food and mucus to create chyme. This mixture then passes into the small intestine.

92. D: Neuromuscular therapy addresses trigger points and their relationship to local and referred pain by using anatomic knowledge and palpatory skills to assess the condition of the tissue and treat neuromuscular lesions. These neuromuscular lesions are often sensitive to pressure and are affiliated with trigger points. The treatment normalizes the tissue and breaks the cycle of pain and dysfunction.

93. A: The anterior fibers of the deltoid muscle originate on the lateral one-third of the clavicle and insert into the deltoid tuberosity of the humerus.

94. C: The lumbar plexus is formed by the first four of the five lumbar nerves. These nerves supply the skin, the abdominal organs, and the hip, knee, leg, and thigh. The femoral and obturator nerves are part of the lumbar plexus.

95. D: A dual relationship is a relationship that consists of both a therapeutic relationship between the practitioner and client as well as a secondary relationship that is outside of the normal therapeutic environment.

96. C: The antagonist is the muscle that opposes the prime mover. The antagonist must perform the opposite action of the prime mover to allow the movement to happen. For example, when lifting a cup, the biceps will contract to perform the movement, whereas the triceps lengthen and extend in the opposing direction to allow the movement.

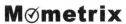

97. A: The three normal end feels are hard, soft, and springy. A hard end feel is one that is abrupt and painless and feels like bone on bone. A soft end feel is one where soft tissue prevents any further movement. A springy end feel is created by the stretch of fibrous tissue at the end of the range of motion.

98. D: Tylenol is classified as a non-opioid analgesic. It is sold over the counter and is used to relieve mild to moderate pain, fever, and some inflammatory conditions like arthritis. Non-opioid analgesics are not considered habit-forming and do not cause withdrawal symptoms.

99. C: Transference happens in a therapeutic relationship when a client personalizes the relationship and begins to unconsciously project characteristics of someone from a previous relationship onto the practitioner. The client may have misperceptions regarding the intent of the relationship. Signs of transference include the giving of gifts, asking personal questions, and attempts to befriend the practitioner.

100. A: If a client has already been referred by a physician and no injury was found, the practitioner should reassess the client and evaluate whether the treatment plan is effective. If the practitioner creates a new treatment plan that does not show results after a few sessions, then the client should return to the original physician for follow-up care.

MBLEx Practice Test #2

1. Which three classes of lymphocytes circulate in the bloodstream?

    a. Cytotoxic T cells, stromal cells, and plasma cells

    b. B cells, NK cells, and stromal cells

    c. Cytotoxic T cells, helper T cells, and suppressor T cells

    d. Thymus-dependent T cells, bone marrow-derived B cells, and natural killer cells

2. When friction is applied to the skin, it increases the dissipation of heat by approximately ___.

    a. 60%

    b. 75%

    c. 80%

    d. 95%

3. What is the primary function of antidiuretic hormone (ADH)?

    a. It stimulates cell growth and replication.

    b. It increases production of melanocytes in the skin.

    c. It decreases the amount of water lost from the kidneys.

    d. It stimulates smooth muscle contractions in the wall of the uterus.

4. A synovial joint that allows one bone to rotate around the surface of another bone is called a(an):

    a. gliding joint.

    b. pivot joint.

    c. saddle joint.

    d. ellipsoid joint.

5. In cross-fiber friction, the direction of the stroke is applied:

    a. transversely.

    b. longitudinally.

    c. circularly.

    d. medially.

6. Which of the following is NOT a form of depression?

    a. Bipolar disorder

    b. Posttraumatic stress disorder

    c. Seasonal affective disorder

    d. Dysthymic disorder

7. Which is the best definition of wellness?

    a. A measure of how healthy an individual is.

    b. A response to being healthful.

    c. Behaviors and habits that have a positive influence on health.

    d. Behaviors that positively affect health.

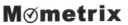

8. How many phalanges do each of the second through fifth toes contain?

    a. 1
    b. 2
    c. 3
    d. 4

9. Which type of data is obtained through assessment by palpation?

    a. Objective
    b. Subjective
    c. Neither
    d. Both

10. Which muscles of the forearm make up the "wad of three?"

    a. Brachioradialis, extensor carpi radialis longus, extensor carpi radialis brevis
    b. Extensor indicis, extensor digitorum, extensor retinaculum
    c. Brachioradialis, anconeus, extensor carpi ulnaris
    d. Extensor carpi ulnaris, extensor digitorum, extensor digiti minimi

11. A client is experiencing pain related to exacerbation of rheumatoid arthritis and has requested a massage. Is massage during this period safe for the client?

    a. Yes, as long as the client communicates her level of pain tolerance.
    b. Yes, because gentle massage can reduce stress and provide comfort.
    c. No, massage will worsen any inflammation during this period.
    d. No, massage is not safe for individuals with RA either during symptom exacerbation or remission.

12. Which of the following is NOT an example of dry heat?

    a. Heating pad
    b. Infrared radiation
    c. Microwave
    d. Sauna

13. Which cranial nerve innervates the lateral rectus muscle?

    a. Abducens
    b. Oculomotor
    c. Vestibulocochlear
    d. Vagus

14. Which phase is part of mitosis?

    a. G1 phase
    b. G2 phase
    c. S phase
    d. Metaphase

15. Which of the following is a way to personalize the connection between a therapist and a client?

a. Maintaining eye contact
b. Using the client's name
c. Listening attentively during the consultation
d. All of the above

16. What is "touch for health?"

a. Another term for massage
b. A form of applied kinesiology
c. A specific type of passive touch
d. A program developed out of structural integration

17. The action of the pectoralis major muscle is:

a. adduction and flexion at the shoulder.
b. flexion, adduction, and medial rotation at the shoulder.
c. extension, adduction, and medial rotation at the shoulder.
d. depression and protraction of the shoulder.

18. At which step in the contraction cycle does the power stroke occur?

a. The formation of cross-bridges
b. The detachment of cross-bridges
c. The pivoting of myosin heads
d. The reactivation of myosin heads

19. Which of the following are classified as types of pain responses?

a. Psychological and physical
b. Physiological and physical
c. Psychological and physiological
d. Physical and anatomical

20. Which of the following involves protrusion of the nucleus pulposus through a tear in the annulus fibrosus?

a. Slipped disc
b. Ruptured disc
c. Herniated disc
d. Bulging disc

21. A(n) _____ contraction occurs when the peak tension developed in a muscle is less than the load and the muscle elongates.

a. concentric
b. eccentric
c. isometric
d. egocentric

22. When writing a SOAP note, what information should be included in the "objective" portion?

  a. Techniques used during the session and any changes in the client's symptoms.
  b. Suggestions for future sessions.
  c. Information gathered by the therapist during history taking, observation, and interview.
  d. Anything the client tells the therapist.

23. What is the most appropriate massage to be done on an area affected by lymphedema?

  a. Superficial friction
  b. Lymph drainage
  c. Derivative massage
  d. Passive touch

24. Friction is being applied _____ if the movement is in the same direction of the blood flow in the veins.

  a. centripetally
  b. centrifugally
  c. distally
  d. proximally

25. How long can you apply friction to dry skin?

  a. 3-6 minutes
  b. 4-7 minutes
  c. 5-8 minutes
  d. 6-9 minutes

26. Which of the following is an example of an effect of massage on the muscular system?

  a. Heightens blood circulation to the skin.
  b. Favorably influences organs of the body.
  c. Increases activity of sudoriferous and sebaceous glands.
  d. Positively affects the range of motion of limbs that have limited range due to tissue injury.

27. What is NOT included in the marketing portion of a business plan?

  a. Clarified differential advantage
  b. Risk assessment
  c. Competition analysis
  d. Budget

28. Which of the following is a therapeutic application of deep kneading?

  a. Relieving the cold that arises from spasms of the small vessels.
  b. Promoting absorption in instances of serous effusion into the pleural cavity.
  c. Increasing weak muscles in size and firmness.
  d. A and B.

29. **Which of the following components of bone is made up of outer fibrous and inner cellular layers?**
    a. Canaliculi
    b. Periosteum
    c. Matrix
    d. Osteocytes

30. **How much of your work time should be invested in marketing?**
    a. 25%
    b. 20%
    c. 15%
    d. 10%

31. **Which of the following statements best describes collagen fibers?**
    a. They permit stretching and then recoil to their original length.
    b. They resist stretching but are easily bent or twisted.
    c. They do not permit stretching but will recoil to original length.
    d. They resist stretching and are not easily bent or twisted.

32. **There is evidence that massage was employed by the Chinese as early as ____ years ago.**
    a. 2000
    b. 2500
    c. 3000
    d. 3500

33. **The kidneys rely on three distinct processes to perform their functions. They are:**
    a. diffusion, osmosis, and carrier-mediated transport.
    b. filtration, reabsorption, and secretion.
    c. absorption, secretion, and reabsorption.
    d. filtration, collection, and channel-mediated diffusion.

34. **Wellness is often represented as an equilateral triangle with three aspects that a wellness-oriented person strives to attain. Those three sides that the wellness model depicts are:**
    a. psychological, mental, and mindful.
    b. emotions, attitude, and spirit.
    c. conditions, situations, and practices.
    d. physical, psychological/mental, and attitude/emotional.

35. **What does light stroking do?**
    a. Causes a contraction of the blood vessels
    b. Hastens the flow of blood through the superficial veins
    c. Enhances lymph flow
    d. Dilates the capillaries

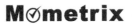

36. Which of the following is a reason why it can be challenging for therapists to give high-quality therapeutic massage in a spa setting?

a. Low expectations from spa guests
b. Time constraints
c. Inexperienced clients who have not formed an appreciation for bodywork
d. All of the above

37. Which explanation best describes the first metatarsal?

a. It is long and slender
b. Its dorsal and medial sides are deep and difficult to palpate
c. It articulates with the medial cuneiform
d. It is an attachment site for the peroneus brevis

38. Kyphosis is an exaggerated curvature of:

a. the cervical spine.
b. the thoracic spine.
c. the lumbar spine.
d. each portion of the spine at once.

39. When preparing stones for a hot stone massage, water in the heating container should be kept between which temperatures?

a. 100° and 130°F
b. 110° and 140°F
c. 120° and 150°F
d. 130° and 160°F

40. In pétrissage, the muscles should be lifted from the bone or underlying tissue from what point?

a. The point of insertion
b. The point of origin
c. The most lateral point
d. The most proximal point

41. What does a release of information form contain?

a. The client's name and the therapist's name
b. The client's name and the name of the person(s) the information is being given to
c. The client's name and the time frame in which the information may be released
d. The client's name, the therapist's name, the name of the person(s) the information is being given to, and the time frame in which the information may be released

42. Which type of gland secretes the "fight or flight" hormones?

a. Pituitary
b. Adrenal
c. Exocrine
d. Endocrine

43. What is pathology?
   a. The study of viruses
   b. The study of disease
   c. The study of pain
   d. The study of structure

44. Contraindications that require the practitioner to adjust the massage when there are health concerns that render certain techniques inadvisable are called:
   a. regional contraindications.
   b. conditional contraindications.
   c. partial contraindications.
   d. absolute contraindications.

45. What is the Swedish system of massage primarily based on?
   a. Shiatsu, a finger pressure method
   b. Chi, the life force energy
   c. Western concepts of anatomy and physiology
   d. Various kinds of therapeutic baths

46. The vein and lymph channels are ____ in the vicinity of the ____.
   a. larger, joints
   b. smaller, joints
   c. larger, limbs
   d. smaller, limbs

47. Which kind of bath should be at a temperature of 90° to 94°F to stimulate circulation?
   a. Hot bath
   b. Warm bath
   c. Saline bath
   d. Tepid bath

48. Skeletal muscle is composed of all of the following except:
   a. fascia.
   b. nerves.
   c. osteocytes.
   d. blood vessels.

49. What role does a muscle play if it carries out an action?
   a. Agonist
   b. Synergist
   c. Antagonist
   d. Protagonist

50. Which technique can powerfully stimulate the nutrition of a joint?
   a. Beating
   b. Active touch
   c. Deep vibration
   d. Stretching

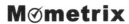

51. Which early advocate of massage discovered that sleep may be induced by gentle stroking?

    a. Hippocrates
    b. Asclepiads
    c. Herodicus
    d. Plutarch

52. Which of the following rules is false in regards to abdominal massage?

    a. General abdominal massage should not be administered until two hours after eating.
    b. The bladder should be emptied just before abdominal massage.
    c. Superficial movements should be avoided at first when working with a "ticklish" patient.
    d. Deep-kneading movements should be applied more quickly than for other parts of the body.

53. Which option includes the structures of concern for the endangerment site that is at the anterior triangle of the neck?

    a. Brachial plexus, subclavian artery, brachiocephalic vein, external jugular vein, and lymph nodes
    b. Axillary, median, musculocutaneous and ulnar nerves; axillary artery, axillary nerve, and lymph nerves
    c. Carotid artery, internal jugular vein, vagus nerve, and lymph nodes
    d. Median nerve, radial and ulnar arteries, and median cubital vein

54. Which gastrointestinal condition is characterized by abnormal muscular contractions?

    a. Crohn's disease
    b. Irritable bowel syndrome
    c. Ulcerative colitis
    d. Diverticulitis

55. What year was sports massage introduced into the Olympics?

    a. 1964
    b. 1974
    c. 1984
    d. 1994

56. What does "phagocytosis" literally mean?

    a. Cell drinking
    b. Cell eating
    c. Cell excreting
    d. Cell secreting

57. Which of the following is not an effect of the positive touch of massage?

    a. Lowered cortisol levels
    b. Lowered norepinephrine levels
    c. Lowered stress levels
    d. Lowered serotonin and dopamine levels

58. Is certification from a state or municipal regulating agency issued in the same way a license is issued?

a. Yes, a certification and a license are the same thing.
b. Yes, it just depends on what a particular state prefers to call it.
c. No, a certification is not as valid as a license.
d. No, a certification is awarded by schools, institutions, and professional organizations.

59. When is the observation portion of a client assessment?

a. From the moment the client walks in the door until the client leaves.
b. From when the initial interview begins to when it ends.
c. From when the initial interview begins to when the treatment ends.
d. From the moment the client walks in the door to the end of the initial interview.

60. What do beta-blockers do?

a. Decrease blood pressure
b. Affect heart rate
c. Affect the strength of contractions
d. All of the above

61. Which of the following is an example of someone who would be considered an independent contractor?

a. A massage therapist who is told what fee to charge her clients.
b. A massage therapist who performs her services under given guidelines.
c. A massage therapist who is reimbursed for business and travel expenses.
d. A massage therapist who is paid directly by her clients.

62. What is kinesiology?

a. The scientific study of muscular activity and mechanics of body movement.
b. The study of the structural and functional changes caused by disease.
c. The study of the gross structure of the body.
d. The science and study of the vital processes, mechanisms, and functions of an organ or system of organs.

63. To practice good ethics is to be concerned about all of the following except:

a. the public welfare.
b. your own welfare.
c. the welfare of individual clients.
d. the reputation of the profession you represent.

64. Which of the following is NOT a major fee-setting strategy?

a. Setting a high price to target a small percentage of the population.
b. Setting a price that competes with the going rate for the industry.
c. Setting a lower price to gain a larger share of the market.
d. All of the above are fee-setting strategies.

65. What does relationship-based marketing involve?

a. Getting relatives to refer their friends and family to you.
b. Getting clients to refer family members to you.
c. Truly caring about your clients' welfare.
d. Hiring a spouse for PR to help you expand your client base.

66. Who was the innovator of the seated massage, also referred to as chair massage?

a. John Harvey Kellogg
b. David Palmer
c. William Harvey
d. Elizabeth Dicke

67. Which of the following is NOT a major purpose for keeping client files?

a. Future contact when in need of referrals
b. Record keeping and the IRS
c. Keeping well-informed of your client's needs
d. Insurance reimbursement

68. Pain described as "persistent or intermittent over a long period of time, often dull and diffused" is what type of pain?

a. Referred
b. Subtle
c. Acute
d. Chronic

69. Which type of end feel is due to the stretch of fibrous tissue as the joint reaches the extent of its range of motion?

a. Taut end feel
b. Springy end feel
c. Hard end feel
d. Soft end feel

70. Does a client ever sign an informed consent after the initial consultation?

a. No, just during the initial consultation.
b. No, in some places it is not even necessary.
c. Yes, after every few sessions.
d. Yes, when an updated plan is created.

71. Which of the following is a non-steroidal anti-inflammatory drug (NSAID)?

a. Naproxen
b. Celecoxib
c. Cortisone
d. Both A and B

72. If a client tries to sexualize a therapy session, is it appropriate to terminate the session?

 a. Yes, you should walk out without saying anything.
 b. Yes, but you should still plan on maintaining the therapeutic relationship.
 c. Yes, ask the client to dress and leave, then promptly leave the room.
 d. Yes, state that you are uncomfortable, ask the client to dress and leave, and then promptly leave the room.

73. What is innervation?

 a. The distribution of nerves to a region or organ.
 b. A response to stimulation by sensory neurons that are normally inactive.
 c. The synaptic surface where neurotransmitter release occurs.
 d. The reflex in which interneurons are interposed between the sensory fiber and the motor neuron(s).

74. Which of the following types of cancer originates in epithelial tissue?

 a. Sarcoma
 b. Lymphoma
 c. Myeloma
 d. Carcinoma

75. Which business name is the best example for establishing a good reputation?

 a. "Smitty's Massage Parlor"
 b. "Smith Massage Clinic"
 c. Neither A nor B.
 d. Both A and B.

76. If your business plan is going to be used to secure a loan, what additional information should be added that is not otherwise included?

 a. Cover page
 b. Table of contents
 c. Appendix
 d. References

77. Is it a national requirement for massage therapists to be licensed in the United States?

 a. No, only the continental United States.
 b. No, it varies from state to state.
 c. Yes, but the license requirements vary from state to state.
 d. Yes, all the license requirements are the same in each state.

78. In which of the four major client-interview stages do you discuss the client's general issues and expectations?

 a. The initiation stage
 b. The exploration stage
 c. The planning stage
 d. The closing stage

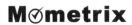

79. All of the following are disadvantages of sole proprietorship except:

    a. All business debts and liabilities are the personal responsibility of the owner.

    b. The therapist possesses the profits.

    c. The owner is responsible for all business aspects.

    d. It may be difficult to obtain financing and unlimited liability.

80. Which is the correct order of the four-part method for resolving an ethical dilemma?

    a. Clarify the problem, identify the problem, describe what action should be taken, identify who should take action.

    b. Identify the problem, clarify the problem, describe what action should be taken, identify who should take action.

    c. Identify who should take action, identify the problem, clarify the problem, describe what action should be taken.

    d. Identify who should take action, identify the problem, describe what action should be taken, clarify the problem.

81. What type of barrier is the first sign of resistance to movement as tissue is manipulated through its range of motion?

    a. Soft tissue barrier

    b. Resistive barrier

    c. Physiologic barrier

    d. Anatomical barrier

82. A client is considered ____ during a massage session due to the inherent nature of the practitioner/client relationship.

    a. timid

    b. shy

    c. vulnerable

    d. quiet

83. How many hours after the injury occurred is local massage contraindicated for whiplash?

    a. 48

    b. 72

    c. 96

    d. Massage would be beneficial immediately following a whiplash injury.

84. Which structure contains densely packed myofibrils, large glycogen reserves, and relatively few mitochondria?

    a. White muscles

    b. Red muscles

    c. Fast fibers

    d. Slow fibers

85. Which of the following is classified as a diverse group of organisms that are potentially capable of causing disease?

    a. Cocci

    b. Bacilli

    c. Spirilla

    d. Fungi

86. An individual's scope of practice is directly related to ____.

a. the skills she has gained and the training she has received.
b. the rights and activities that are acceptable.
c. the styles and techniques that she studied.
d. whether or not she lives in a state that has adopted licensing regulations governing the practice of massage.

87. What does "interpersonal space" refer to?

a. The actual space maintained between the client and practitioner during interactions before and after the massage.
b. The space maintained between the client and practitioner during the actual massage.
c. The amount of space present in any height differences between the client and the practitioner.
d. The minimum amount of space required for a client to feel that the practitioner is being fully attentive.

88. Is it acceptable, as a massage therapist, to sell products in your business?

a. Yes, you can sell anything.
b. Yes, you can sell health care related products.
c. No, you have to be a doctor, nutritionist, or herbologist.
d. No, you're not allowed to sell products in a massage clinic setting.

89. Fibrous tissues that have tensions placed on them during muscular contractions are called:

a. ligaments.
b. cartilage.
c. contractile tissues.
d. striated muscle fibers.

90. Due to the nature of chair massage, which of the following techniques is NOT appropriate?

a. Deep touch
b. Percussion
c. Friction
d. Effleurage

91. Long, relaxing massages affect the autonomic nervous system by ____ the sympathetic nervous system and ____ the parasympathetic nervous system.

a. stimulating, sedating
b. sedating, stimulating
c. stimulating, stimulating
d. sedating, sedating

92. Which is NOT an example of a stimulating massage technique?

a. Pétrissage
b. Friction
c. Percussion
d. Vibration

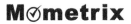

93. Which of the following is essential to keep in mind about personal business cards?

    a. Keep a substantial quantity and always have some with you.
    b. Beauty is in simplicity of design.
    c. Convey major benefits in a quick glance.
    d. All of the above.

94. When assessing passive movement, pain and limitation in all directions generally indicate:

    a. bursitis.
    b. stretching of involved tissues.
    c. compressing of involved tissues.
    d. capsulitis.

95. All of the following are reasons that a license may be revoked, suspended, or canceled except:

    a. having a history of felony conviction.
    b. engaging in any act of prostitution.
    c. having too many speeding tickets in a certain amount of time.
    d. being guilty of fraudulent or deceptive advertising.

96. The resting tension in a skeletal muscle is called:

    a. muscle tone.
    b. muscle contraction.
    c. muscle tension.
    d. motor unit.

97. Which of the following correctly defines the acronym TART?

    a. Tautness, asymmetry, range of motion, tenderness
    b. Texture, asymmetry, range of motion, tenderness
    c. Tautness, active range of motion, range of motion, tenderness
    d. Texture, active range of motion, range of motion, tautness

98. In which of the four major client-interview stages do you create a vision with your client about his major goals?

    a. The initiation stage
    b. The exploration stage
    c. The planning stage
    d. The closure stage

99. Why are licenses and permits required?

    a. To raise revenue.
    b. To protect the health and safety of the public.
    c. Neither A nor B.
    d. Both A and B.

100. When a force is applied between the resistance and the fulcrum, which class of levers is it considered to be?

 a. First-class lever
 b. Second-class lever
 c. Third-class lever
 d. All of the above

101. In Swedish massage, you should always massage in which direction?

 a. Toward the heart.
 b. Away from the heart.
 c. Downward along the limbs.
 d. Centrifugally.

102. Is massage ever indicated during pregnancy, as long as there are not any extenuating circumstances that would otherwise be contraindicated?

 a. Yes, after the first trimester.
 b. Yes, after the second trimester.
 c. Yes, after the third trimester.
 d. Yes, during any trimester.

103. In most organs, _____ reflexes are most important in regulating visceral activities.

 a. long
 b. short
 c. cranial
 d. visceral

104. Which of the following correctly defines kinetic energy?

 a. Energy that has the potential to do work.
 b. Energy that has the capacity to perform work.
 c. The movement of an object.
 d. Energy that is doing work.

105. What is homeostasis?

 a. The internal balance of the body.
 b. The life-force of the body.
 c. An indication of disease.
 d. A condition that causes stress or strain.

106. Which of the following best defines a chronic inflammatory skin disorder where the proliferation rate of epidermal cells is accelerated?

 a. Atopic dermatitis
 b. Eczematous dermatitis
 c. Psoriasis
 d. Seborrhea

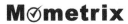

107. What does the brain stem include?

a. Cerebrum, gyri, sulci
b. Mesencephalon, pons, medulla oblongata
c. Cerebrum, pons, medulla oblongata
d. Mesencephalon, gyri, sulci

108. What is countertransference?

a. When a client tries to personalize the therapeutic relationship.
b. When a client tries to de-personalize the therapeutic relationship.
c. When a practitioner tries to personalize the therapeutic relationship.
d. When a practitioner tries to de-personalize the therapeutic relationship.

109. Which of the following are the three most common learning styles among people?

a. Visual, auditory, tactile
b. Visual, tactile, aesthetic
c. Auditory, kinesthetic, solitary
d. Visual, auditory, kinesthetic

110. Which of the following refers to the proportional limitation of a joint that is controlled by muscular contractions?

a. Capsular pattern
b. Hard end feel
c. Soft end feel
d. Contractile tissue

111. Is massage indicated or contraindicated for a client with gout?

a. Massage is indicated during and between gout attacks.
b. Massage is indicated only between gout attacks.
c. Massage is always contraindicated during a gout attack, but is indicated between attacks.
d. Massage is contraindicated during and between gout attacks.

112. What is the 5th cranial nerve?

a. Oculomotor
b. Trochlear
c. Trigeminal
d. Facial

113. Which of the following is a common disinfectant that is found in everyday use?

a. Chlorine bleach
b. Ethyl
c. Cresol
d. All of the above

114. How can massage be helpful for a client with angina pectoris?

a. It reduces stress
b. It decreases the effects of the sympathetic nervous system
c. Both A and B
d. Neither A nor B

115. What does friction do?

a. It increases the permeability of the capillary beds
b. It increases the amount of blood stores in the muscles
c. It stimulates the flow of blood through the deeper arteries and veins
d. It reduces lymphedema

116. Which barrier represents the extent of easy movement allowed during range of motion?

a. Soft tissue
b. Resistive
c. Physiologic
d. Anatomical

117. Which of the following is a mechanical effect of friction?

a. Increased phagocytosis
b. Reduced cerebral congestion
c. Decreased inflammation
d. Improved "hidebound" skins

118. Which of the following is considered a dual relationship?

a. A person who also happens to be a massage therapist becomes a client.
b. A client makes advances towards the practitioner.
c. A family member becomes a client.
d. Any therapeutic relationship between the client and the massage practitioner.

119. Why is it better to pay monthly business bills with a business check?

a. It provides better documentation than cash.
b. It is considered more legitimate than cash.
c. You shouldn't use a business check; you should pay with cash.
d. You shouldn't use a business check; you should use a personal check.

120. Which of the following is one of the major contraindications to consider before administering massage?

a. Abnormal body temperature
b. Acute infectious disease
c. Inflammation
d. All of the above

121. The term used to observe the manner in which a person walks to determine constrictions or related conditions is called:

a. gait.
b. gait assessment.
c. posture assessment.
d. observation.

122. Which of the following is not a type of boundary?

a. Professional
b. Personal
c. Ethical
d. Intellectual

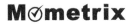

123. At what point is massage appropriate on a client who has meningitis?

   a. Immediately, to help decrease inflammation of the meninges more quickly.
   b. When inflammation of the meninges has begun to subside.
   c. Not until the patient is cleared from the hospital.
   d. Never, it is postponed until the client is completely healed.

124. Which theory proves the example of briskly rubbing a part of the body that has been struck by an object to relieve the intensity of pain?

   a. Endorphin theory
   b. Nociceptor theory
   c. Gate control theory
   d. Superficial friction theory

125. Which glands secrete a watery solution that contains enzymes?

   a. Mixed exocrine glands
   b. Exocrine glands
   c. Serous glands
   d. Mucous glands

Answer Key and Explanations for Test #2

1. D: The three classes of lymphocytes that circulate in blood are thymus-dependent T cells, bone marrow-derived B cells, and NK (natural killer) cells. T cells make up approximately 80% of circulating lymphocytes, while B cells make up 10-15%, and the remaining 5-10% is made up of NK cells.

2. D: Friction raises skin temperature by bringing more blood to the surface, thereby increasing the production of heat. This causes a 95% increase in heat dissipation. Friction encourages circulation by accelerating the flow of the blood and the lymph by emptying the veins, lymph spaces, and channels.

3. C: The primary function of ADH is to control how much water is lost through the kidneys. With the loss minimized, water absorbed from the digestive tract will be retained, which reduces the concentrations of electrolytes in the extracellular fluid. ADH release is inhibited by alcohol, which is why there is an increase in fluid excretion after consuming alcoholic beverages.

4. B: A pivot joint is a type of synovial joint that allows one bone to rotate around the surface of another bone. Synovial joints contain a joint cavity, which is the space that allows for six different types of movement. An example of a pivot joint is the atlantoaxial joint between C1 and C2; this joint allows for rotation of the head.

5. A: Cross-fiber friction is applied with the tips of the fingers or the thumb in a transverse direction across the muscle, tendon, or ligament fibers. Transverse friction is a preferable technique for rehabilitation of fibrous tissue injuries. When healing, transverse friction can promote the formation of elastic fibrous tissue and reduce the formation of fibrosis and scar tissue. This allows the healed injury to retain its original strength and liability.

6. B: Posttraumatic stress disorder is not a form of depression, but is a delayed response of intense anxiety. Some forms of depression include major depressive disorder, bipolar disorder, dysthymic disorder, postpartum depression, and seasonal affective disorder (SAD). Depression is classified as a mood or an affective disorder.

7. C: The best definition of wellness is the behaviors and habits that have a positive influence on health. It is a concept where a person takes responsibility for his state of health and makes an effort to recognize conditions, situations, and practices that may be detrimental to a healthy state. Wellness considers psychological, physical, and emotional health.

8. C: Phalanges are the small bones that make up the fingers and toes. Each finger and each toe contains three phalanges.

9. D: Assessment by palpation is both objective and subjective. Many therapists use palpation as the primary form of assessment, but it is most accurate when used in conjunction with other assessment skills. For example, with a painful condition where the pain is radiating or referred; observation and examination isolate the cause of the pain and then palpation pinpoints the source.

10. A: The brachioradialis, extensor carpi radialis longus, and extensor carpi radialis brevis all form a long mass of muscle that extends distally from the lateral supracondylar ridge of the humerus, collectively known as the "wad of three." It is just lateral to the inner elbow.

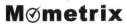

11. C: Massage is contraindicated during an exacerbation period of rheumatoid arthritis because it will worsen the inflammation that is present. When in remission, it is safe to administer massage to a client with RA. Areas and nodules that are tender should be avoided. The massage can reduce stress and gentle stretches and joint mobilizations can help increase joint mobility.

12. C: A heating pad, infrared radiation, and a sauna are all examples of dry heat. A microwave as well as a shortwave, are examples of diathermy. Diathermy is the application of oscillating electromagnetic fields to the tissue; this causes a distortion in the molecules and an ionic vibration that produces heat. Its use requires special equipment and training, and it is beyond the scope of practice of a massage therapist.

13. A: The lateral rectus muscle is innervated by the abducens nerves (VI). This pair of nerves originates in the pons and passes through the superior orbital fissures of the sphenoid bone. They are the sixth pair of extra-ocular muscles and essentially cause abduction of the eye.

14. D: Metaphase is the second stage of mitosis, which begins as the chromatids move to a narrow central zone that is called the metaphase plate. When all of the chromatids are aligned in the plane of the metaphase plate, the metaphase ends.

15. D: Maintaining visual contact, using the client's name when speaking with them, and listening attentively during the consultation are all ways of personalizing the connection between a therapist and the client. Mirroring the client's body language, voice tone, and language can also build rapport. Good rapport is the basis for trust, mutual respect, and openness that can enhance a therapeutic relationship.

16. B: Touch for health is a simplified form of applied kinesiology. Its methods are derived from both Eastern and Western origins. The purpose of this technique is to relieve stress on muscles and internal organs. Kinesiology is the principle of anatomy in relation to human movement and was developed by Dr. John Thie, D.C.

17. B: The pectoralis major muscle extends between the anterior portion of the chest and the crest of the greater tubercle of the humerus. When working on its own, it produces flexion at the shoulder joint. When working with the latissimus dorsi, it produces adduction and medial rotation of the humerus at the shoulder.

18. C: The power stroke occurs after the cross-bridge formation, during the pivoting of myosin heads. The energy to cock the myosin head is obtained by breaking down ATP into ADP and a phosphate group. In this position, the ADP and the phosphate are still bound to the myosin head. After the formation of cross-bridges, stored energy is released as the myosin head pivots toward the M line. This action is called the power stroke.

19. A: Two types of responses to pain are psychological and physical. The physical response to pain is characterized by an increase in blood pressure and pulse, and a shift in blood flow to the muscles. The psychological reaction to pain is characterized by fear, anxiety, tension, and fatigue.

20. C: A herniated disc is a protrusion of the nucleus pulposus through a tear in the annulus fibrosus. This tear can occur at the time of trauma or it can develop gradually after the trauma. This protrusion can exert pressure on the spinal nerve roots, causing pain that radiates along the path of the compressed nerve.

21. B: There are two types of isotonic contractions: concentric and eccentric. When an eccentric contraction occurs, the peak tension developed is less than the load, and the muscle elongates due

191

to the contraction of another muscle or the pull of gravity. Eccentric contractions are common and are involved in a variety of movements.

22. C: The "objective" portion of a SOAP note includes any information gathered by the therapist during history taking, observation, and interview, as well as assessment procedures and tests. The therapist's treatment goals are also noted. Information from this objective assessment as well as data from the subjective assessment is used to design the massage session.

23. B: Lymphedema usually affects an extremity; it happens when interstitial fluid accumulates or swelling occurs in the soft tissues due to inflammation, blockage, or removal of the lymph channels. Lymphedema occurs when fluid accumulates in the interstitial spaces because it cannot pass into or through the lymph channels. A lymph drainage massage promotes the drainage of fluid accumulation.

24. A: Friction is being applied centripetally if the movement is in the same direction of the veins. The movement comes from below and travels upward; going from the hands and feet toward the body and using the thumb or palmar surface of the hand. The amount of pressure applied when utilizing friction should not be so little that the hand slips over the surface, or so great that it interferes with the movement of the blood in the arteries.

25. C: 5-8 minutes is as long as it is safe to apply friction to dry skin. It is important to take notice that skin does not become irritated by working too long without lubrication. Friction without lubrication would be effective when using the reflex effect in cases where peripheral circulation is less than optimal.

26. D: Along with increasing range of motion, massage stimulates circulation, nerve supply, and cell activity. It can also relax tense muscles and release muscle spasms. Massage can prevent or relieve stiffness and soreness of muscles and decrease the time needed to restore muscles that have been fatigued by work or exercise. The other options listed are physiological effects of massage to the skin and viscera.

27. B: Risk assessment is part of a business plan but is not included under the marketing section. Things considered when outlining the marketing portion of a business plan are descriptions of target markets and clarifications of differential advantage, a competition analysis, a strategic action plan, a marketing budget, and a summary of how marketing strategies will enable success.

28. C: A therapeutic application of deep kneading is an increase in size and firmness of weak muscles. Deep kneading is a valuable method to use in cases of paralysis and paresis, or in any case where there is tissue weakness and relaxation. Enlarged, stiffened, and painful joints may return to a normal state when inflammation is decreased.

29. B: The periosteum is the substance that covers the outer surfaces of bones. It consists of outer fibrous and inner cellular layers, but does not cover the joints. Other characteristics of bone are the matrix, which is dense and contains calcium salt deposits; osteocytes, which are a kind of bone cells; and canaliculi, which are narrow passageways that form a branching network for exchanging of nutrients, waste products, and gases.

30. C: At least 15% of work time should be invested in marketing. Regular marketing is critical during all phases of owning and running a business, but it is also a practice that most health care practitioners neglect. It is essential to a successful business to not just rely on referrals or to slack on marketing after it is actively established.

31. B: There are two types of fibers that contribute to dermal strength and elasticity. Collagen fibers are very strong; they resist stretching but are easily bent or twisted. On the other hand, elastic fibers permit stretching and recoil to their original length. The collagen fibers limit flexibility to prevent damage to the tissue, but elastic fibers provide the tissue with some mobility.

32. C: Evidence suggests that massage was employed by the Chinese as early as 3000 years ago. It is probably one of the oldest of all forms of relief of illnesses or injuries. An ancient Chinese book called "The Cong-Fou of the Tao-Tse" was probably the foundation of both modern massage as well as the manual Swedish movements. Massage is still used extensively by the Chinese today.

33. B: To perform their functions, the kidneys rely on filtration, reabsorption, and secretion. During filtration, blood pressure forces water and solutes across the wall of the glomerular capillaries and into the capsular space. Then, solute molecules that are small enough to pass through the filtration membrane are carried by the surrounding water molecules. In reabsorption, the water and solutes from the filtrate are removed. They then move across the tubular epithelium and into the peritubular fluid. Secretion is often the primary method of excretion for some compounds; it transports solutes from the peritubular fluid, across the tubular epithelium, and into the tubular fluid.

34. D: The wellness triangle depicts the body, mind, and spirit or the physical, psychological/mental, and attitude/emotional. When all three of these aspects are healthy and in balance, a state of optimum wellness is achieved. This includes maintaining a positive mental and spiritual attitude, reducing health risks, and eliminating practices that add stress or danger to a lifestyle. Wellness is a concept in which a person takes personal responsibility for his state of health and makes an effort to recognize conditions that may be threatening or detrimental to his health.

35. D: Certain massage movements affect the blood and lymph channels in various ways. Light stroking temporarily dilates the capillaries instantaneously. Deep stroking results in a more lasting dilation and flushing of the area being massaged.

36. D: A massage session done in a spa can be as therapeutic as one done elsewhere, but it can also be challenging due to the nature of scheduling and the clients typical of a spa. Spa guests may arrive without any present complaints and do not expect much out of the massage therapy session beyond relaxation. It is also difficult for therapists to retain enthusiasm and high energy levels when under strict time constraints each day. Additionally, inexperienced clients who have not yet been educated about the effects and benefits of massage can contribute to a more challenging therapeutic massage session.

37. C: The proximal end of the first metatarsal articulates with the medial cuneiform. It is short and stocky, not long and slender like the metatarsals of toes two through five. The dorsal and medial sides are superficial and easily accessible, although its plantar surface is deep.

38. B: Kyphosis or hyper-kyphosis is an exaggeration of the normal posterior curvature (20-40 degrees) or an excessive rounding (45-50 degrees) of the thoracic spine. Characteristics of a person affected by kyphosis are a hunchback, and an apparently caved in chest with arms that tend to hang in front of the body. Rounded shoulders and a dowager's hump are also sometimes classified as mild kyphosis.

39. B: The water in the heating container should be kept between 110° and 140°F. Temperatures that are below 110°F will not be sufficiently warm enough for therapeutic application, and temperatures that are above 140°F will be difficult for the client to handle. Stones that are heated beyond this temperature may cause discomfort or even damage to the tissue if applied directly to the skin.

40. A: In pétrissage, the muscles should be lifted from the bone, and rolled and stretched in an upward direction or from the point of insertion. Whenever a muscle is grasped, it should be dragged outward from the median line at the same time. The grasp should then be released when the strain is at its maximum, which will encourage the highest degree of flow of fluids toward the parts being operated on.

41. D: A release of information form contains the client's name, the therapist's name, the name of the person(s) the information is being given to, and the time frame in which the information may be released. Files and information about the client are kept confidential unless pertinent data is being shared with the client's insurance company or other health professionals who are caring for the client. At this point, the information is only released when appropriate release of information forms have been properly signed. The completed form is signed, dated, and kept in the client's file. The only other time information from a client may be given is if it is ordered by a court of law.

42. B: Adrenal glands, which are situated on top of the kidneys, produce epinephrine, norepinephrine, and corticosteroids. These glands create the adrenaline that is most notably associated with the "fight or flight" response. Adrenal secretions give a physical and mental boost that heightens senses, sharpens reflexes, and prepares muscles when encountered with a high level of stress.

43. B: Pathology is the study of disease. Disease is a condition of abnormal function that involves anatomic structures or body systems. Diseases are characterized by signs and symptoms that are recognizable and they are typically attributed to heredity, infection, diet, or environmental factors.

44. B: Conditional contraindications require the practitioner to adjust the massage. Some techniques may cause discomfort or have adverse effects, while other therapeutic applications may still be very beneficial. It is important that the practitioner know when massage is advised and also when it should be avoided, or when specific strokes or movements should not be used. Contraindications that are absolute are not appropriate; regional or partial contraindications prohibit massage only to certain parts of the body.

45. C: The Swedish system of massage is based on the Western concepts of anatomy and physiology. It employs the traditional manipulative techniques such as tapotement, friction, vibration, pétrissage, and effleurage. It also employs additional movements that can be slow and gentle or vigorous and bracing depending on what the practitioner would like to achieve.

46. A: The vein and lymph channels are larger in the vicinity of the joints than in any other part of the limbs. This is due to the great amount of absorption that is required to keep the articulating surfaces in good condition. This is also why joint movement and manipulation is capable of producing powerful derivative effects upon more distal parts.

47. C: A saline or salt bath should be at a temperature of 90° to 94°F and produces a tonic effect achieved by stimulating circulation. The effect of a saline bath is similar to natural bathing in sea water. The typical amount of salt used is 3-5 pounds to a tub of water and the client stays in the bath for 10 to 20 minutes.

48. C: Skeletal muscle does not include osteocytes. It is composed of muscle cells or muscle fibers, layers of connective tissue or fascia, and many nerves and blood vessels. It is the voluntary contractile tissue that moves the skeleton. Some other physical characteristics unique to skeletal muscle tissue are its striated texture, muscle fibers that have direction and can help determine the specific muscle being palpated, and the fact that it can be in a contracted or relaxed state.

49. A: A muscle or group of muscles that carries out an action is called the agonist. A muscle that has an opposite action of the agonist is called an antagonist, while a muscle that supports the agonist is called a synergist. These particular roles played by each muscle or group of muscles are necessary in order for a specific movement to occur.

50. D: Joint stretching is a powerful means of stimulation to a joint. It is a practice employed by the Turks in connection with shampooing during the Turkish bath. Stretching may be applied to the arm and shoulder joints and the finger joints.

51. B: Asclepiads was an eminent Greek physician who discovered that sleep can be induced by gentle stroking. He held the art of massage therapy in such high esteem that he refused the use of medicine of any kind and relied exclusively on massage. He claimed it produced a cure by restoring the nutritive fluids to their natural, free movement.

52. D: Deep-kneading movements should not be applied more quickly during abdominal massage. Deep-kneading movements should be applied more slowly. This allows time for movement of the fecal mass. Additionally, when performing abdominal massage, sudden thrusts should also be avoided which may cause the patient pain. Disturbances that create rigidity of the abdominal muscles will interfere with the effects of the manipulations.

53. C: The endangerment site that is at the anterior triangle of the neck is bordered by the mandible, the sternocleidomastoid muscle, and the trachea. The structures of concern at this site are the carotid artery, internal jugular vein, vagus nerve, and lymph nodes. Endangerment sites are areas of the body that warrant consideration before being massaged due to underlying anatomical structures that can be prone to injury when administering certain manipulations.

54. B: Irritable bowel syndrome (IBS) is a condition of the gastrointestinal system that involves abnormal muscular contractions. It differs from other gastrointestinal diseases in that it does not cause inflammation or any permanent damage to the intestines, nor does it increase the risk of colorectal cancer.

55. C: Massage was introduced to the Summer Olympics in 1984. Since then, sports massage has been included in every Summer and Winter Olympics. Sports massage is a type of massage that is designed to specifically enhance an athlete's performance through specialized manipulations that stimulate circulation of the blood and lymph. A team of sports massage therapists is now a regular sighting at a variety of major sporting events and sought out by many serious athletes.

56. B: Phagocytosis means "cell eating." Most cells display pinocytosis (cell drinking), but phagocytosis is performed by specialized cell-like macrophages that protect tissues by "eating" things such as bacteria, debris, and any other abnormal materials.

57. D: One of the effects of positive touch from massage is an increased level of serotonin and dopamine in the body. This can be significant because low levels of serotonin and dopamine are present in people who suffer from depression, whereas significantly higher levels are present in those with elevated moods. Positive touch can affect human physical and emotional health; it is an essential element for healthy growth and development, as supported by its ability to affect an individual's state of being.

Answer Key and Explanations for Test #2

195

58. D: A certification may be awarded by schools, institutions, or professional organizations to show the successful completion of courses of study or to indicate that certain qualifications have been met. It is a document that is awarded in recognition of an accomplishment or from maintaining some kind of standard. There is a National Certification Board for Therapeutic Massage and Bodywork (NCBTMB); however, it does not take the place of a license where a license is required to practice massage.

59. A: Observation is a major part of the assessment process. Observation begins when the client walks in the door and continues until the client leaves the setting. A key clue to watch for at this stage is the client's body language. It will give insight to where pain and tension are being held, emotional makeup, and self-esteem.

60. D: Beta-blockers are used to treat hypertension and angina pectoris, as well as arrhythmias and migraines. They work by reducing sympathetic arousal and inhibiting the action of catecholamines at beta-adrenergic receptors. They decrease blood pressure, affect heart rate, and affect the strength of the heart's contractions.

61. D: It is important to be sure of someone's status as an independent contractor. If the IRS determines that a person hired as an independent contractor actually qualifies as an employee, you may be required to pay a heavy fine. Some characteristics that are indicative of an independent contractor status are: having the ability to pursue other clients, providing their own supplies, setting their own schedules while working no more than 20 hours per week, and clients paying them directly.

62. A: Kinesiology is the study of muscular activity and the mechanics, physiology, and anatomy of body movement. Other topics that are related to the study of therapeutic massage are anatomy, physiology, histology, and pathology.

63. B: To practice good ethics is to be concerned about your reputation, but not necessarily your own welfare. Ethics are moral guidelines that are established by professionals which aim to reduce the incidence and risk of harm or injury in the professional relationship. Without ethics, there cannot be any true professionalism.

64. D: All of the choices listed are correct. Additionally, if you want to break into a new market, you could offer introductory rates for a limited time (such as reduced rates or two-for-one deals), package deals, or a sliding scale. Before finalizing a fee structure, it is important to consider all of the costs involved in running a business, including fixed costs and amenities.

65. C: Relationship-based marketing involves truly caring about your clients' welfare. You essentially become their partner in wellness. This aspect of a therapist-client relationship is about listening, planning, educating, and being proactive and can pay off tremendously.

66. B: The seated chair massage was introduced in 1985 by David Palmer. It helped make massage more accessible to a wider range of people by making it easier to perform in a number of different places and environments. The therapist was no longer confined by heavy tables, sheets, lubricants, and the necessity for complete privacy.

67. A: The only way to document your work in a service industry is to have client files with rudimentary information included, which serves as record keeping and for the IRS. Files also need to be up to date to best inform you of your client's needs. Also, keeping updated and accurate files are necessary for insurance reimbursement, as most insurance companies will not pay for maintenance care; "reasonable and necessary" is the term used to validate a treatment modality.

68. D: Chronic is a term that refers to a lingering or ongoing condition. It is persistent or intermittent over a long period of time, often dull, diffused, and many times does not have an identifiable cause or source. It can be used to refer to pain or illness. If an illness is chronic, it progresses slowly, is difficult or impossible to remedy; and may last weeks, months, years, or be lifelong.

69. B: End feel is the feeling the therapist senses when passively moving a limb to the limit of its range of motion. The quality of this end feel indicates the presence, type, and severity of lesions in the tissues that are associated with the joint. Springy end feel is the most common; an example of springy end feel is hip flexion or extension.

70. D: Informed consent is an ongoing process. Multiple, regular sessions may require the creation of an updated care plan that includes anticipated outcomes, possible side effects, number and duration of sessions, and specific modalities. When the updated plan is finished, it is again discussed with the client and can then be signed indicating continued informed consent.

71. D: Both naproxen and celecoxib are examples of NSAIDs. NSAIDs are medications that are used most often for pain and inflammation. They have pain-reducing (analgesic) and fever-reducing (antipyretic) qualities due to the inhibition of the synthesis of prostaglandins, which are associated with inflammatory responses.

72. D: If a client tries to sexualize a massage therapy session, whether it be through sexual comments, overt advances, or requests for sexual favors, it is appropriate to state that you are uncomfortable with the comments and intentions made by the client and to terminate the session. You can then instruct the client to dress and leave, and then promptly exit the room. It should be documented what took place and what actions were taken.

73. A: Innervation is the distribution of nerves to a region of the body or a particular organ. There are nerves in the body that control specific muscles or muscle groups. There are cranial nerves that originate in the brain and pass through the foramina of the skull. There are also spinal nerves which connect to the spinal cord and pass through the intervertebral foramina.

74. D: Carcinoma originates in the epithelial tissue that lines the organs and body cavities. Sarcoma originates in supportive and connective tissues such as muscles, cartilage, and bone. Lymphoma originates in the lymphatic tissue while myeloma originates in the bone marrow. Another type of cancer is leukemia, which originates in tissues that form blood cells. The types of cancer are determined by the kind of tissue where the cancer cells originate.

75. B: "Smith Massage Clinic" sounds less suggestive and will be perceived by potential clients in a much different way than "Smitty's Massage Parlor". Other ways to help improve the reputation of your clinic is to keep regular business hours as opposed to late-night hours, and to ensure that proper draping techniques are being used.

76. D: If the business plan is being used to secure a loan, a section titled "references" should be included, which will list all pertinent information regarding your current lending institution and the names, addresses, and phone numbers of your attorney, accountant, and business consultant. Information added to the executive summary portion should include the type of business loan(s) you are seeking and a summary of the proposed use of the funds. The financial analysis portion should specify the loan requirements and the purpose of the loan. A cover page, table of contents, and appendix are already included in a regular business plan.

77. B: It is not a national requirement for massage therapists to be licensed in the United States. Approximately two-thirds of the states require licenses for practicing massage therapy, but the definition, educational requirements, and scope of practice all vary depending on the state. While the majority of states show some basic agreement regarding the need to license massage therapists, there are many differences in defining the purpose, object, procedures, and educational requirements. This results in an undefined scope of practice for massage therapy, although it is still important for massage practitioners to recognize and practice within their legal and professional boundaries.

78. A: In the initiation stage, you introduce yourself, establish rapport, discuss general issues and expectations concerning the client, describe what you can do, and review policies and procedures. This helps improve treatment results and satisfaction by knowing what the client expects from you.

79. B: Possession of profits is actually one of the main advantages of sole proprietorship, along with ease of formation, control of all decisions, and more simple financial record keeping. A major way that a sole proprietorship varies from other business structures (corporation, partnership, LLC) is that you and your business are one entity from a legal standpoint. With this in mind, you cannot be treated as an employee of a business.

80. B: You should first identify the problem to determine if it is truly an ethical problem, then clarify the problem by gathering relevant information and define the specific type of ethical breach. Following those steps, describe what action should be taken by mapping out the best way to resolve the issue and then identify who should take action. Discussing the topic with a colleague or engaging in peer supervision are two methods for clarification.

81. B: The resistive barrier, also called the pathological barrier, is the first sign of resistance to a movement. It is important when assessing and treating soft tissue conditions. It is one of three types of barriers that can be considered when testing range of motion, the other two being a physiologic barrier and an anatomical barrier.

82. C: A practitioner/client relationship exhibits a power differential by its inherent nature. The client seeks the knowledge, skill, and authority from the practitioner's services, putting the practitioner in a place of power to provide actions or services that enhance the well-being of the more vulnerable client. During a session, the client literally looks up to and submits to the manipulations of the practitioner. During the entirety of a session, the practitioner is often active while the client is predominately passive.

83. B: Local massage is contraindicated for 72 hours after an initial injury. Massage would worsen the pain and inflammation present after a whiplash injury. Other symptoms associated with whiplash include headaches, neck pain, limited neck mobility, difficulty swallowing, and pain radiating down the arm.

84. C: Fast fibers, which make up most of the skeletal muscle fibers in the body, are large in diameter and contain densely packed myofibrils, large glycogen reserves, and few mitochondria. Muscles that are dominated by fast fibers produce powerful contractions because the tension from a muscle fiber is directly proportional to the number of myofibrils present.

85. D: Fungi are parasitic organisms that grow in wet or damp environments. They are found mostly on the skin and mucous membranes of humans. Fungal infections such as athlete's foot, ringworm, *Candida*, and vaginal yeast infections tend to resist treatment. Molds and yeasts are also considered fungi.

86. A: "Scope of practice" defines the rights and activities legally acceptable according to the licenses of a particular occupation or profession, and an individual's scope of practice is directly related to the skills she has gained and the training she has received. In addition to particular skills and training, an individual's scope of practice is also influenced by personal limitations like belief systems, personal bias, preferred clientele, physical stature, and endurance. Many occupations and professions, including massage therapy, have national or state regulatory boards that define and enforce adherence to a scope of practice.

87. A: "Interpersonal space" refers to the actual space maintained between the client and practitioner during interactions that take place before and after the actual massage. Creating this appropriate space means maintaining a physical distance that makes both parties feel comfortable. It is important to carry on conversations at eye level whenever possible and to complete most of the conversation before the client lies down on the table. This minimizes the power differential and shows respect and consideration to the client.

88. B: It is acceptable to sell products at your place of business that are designed to assist in pain relief and promote well-being. Ethical sales of products are based on educating your clients about the products and allowing the opportunity to purchase them from you. Only products that you know to be reliable and that are a natural extension of your business are appropriate to sell.

89. C: Contractile tissues are fibrous and have tensions placed on them during muscle contractions. Contractile tissues include muscle tissue, tendons, and muscle attachments. This is one of the core concepts used in assessing range of motion, as developed by Dr. James Cyriax. The other concepts are inert tissues, end feel, and capsular pattern.

90. D: Chair massage is an effective way to introduce massage to a person who may exhibit adverse reactions to touch, and is also suitable for those who may consider traditional Swedish massage too invasive. Due to the nature of chair massage, friction, percussion, and deep touches are the only appropriate techniques. With the client seated in the prone position, the head, neck, shoulders, back, and hips may be the only areas the practitioner can access.

91. B: Long, relaxing massages affect the autonomic nervous system by sedating the sympathetic nervous system and stimulating the parasympathetic nervous system. This results in reduced blood levels of epinephrine and norepinephrine, reduced heart rate and blood pressure, and an increased relaxation response.

92. A: Pétrissage is not a type of stimulating massage. Examples of stimulating massage techniques are vibration, which stimulates the peripheral nerves and nerve centers; percussion, which increases nervous irritability (strong percussion for a short period excites nerve centers directly while prolonged percussion anesthetizes local nerves); and friction, which stimulates nerves.

93. D: All of the above options are true. You should always carry a lot of business cards with you wherever you go and keep extras in your car or purse. You should be generous with your promotional materials in order to best circulate them; always hand out at least three business cards per person. You should also keep the card simple and not turn it into a brochure. Business cards must appeal to your target market. An effective card will convey the major benefits in a quick glace so that the client is not overwhelmed by the amount of information.

94. D: When assessing passive movement, pain and limitation in all directions usually involves the whole joint and indicate capsulitis or arthritis. Passive movement findings such as this one indicates the condition of the inert or non-contractile tissues. Limitation and pain at this point are an indication of some sort of dysfunction.

95. C: The number of speeding tickets acquired does not affect a massage practitioner's licensing status. Other reasons that can affect a license being revoked, canceled, or suspended are: being guilty of fraud or deceit in obtaining a license; practicing under a false or assumed name; being addicted to narcotics, alcohol, or other substances that interfere with duties; being willfully negligent in the practice of massage so as to endanger the health of a client; prescribing drugs or medicines without a physician's license, and ethical or sexual misconduct with a client.

96. A: In skeletal muscles, some of the motor units are constantly active, even when the muscle itself is not contracting. These contractions do not produce enough tension to cause movement, but do tense and firm the muscle. The resulting resting tension in a skeletal muscle is called muscle tone. If a muscle has little muscle tone, it appears limp and flaccid. If a muscle has moderate muscle tone, it appears firm and solid.

97. B: The acronym TART stands for texture, asymmetry, range of motion, and tenderness. Texture describes the feel of superficial and deep tissues, which may include taut bands, adherent tissue, hypertonic tissues, or flaccid tissues. Asymmetry in body structure is observed by a rotation, a curve, or a bilateral inconsistency in the body structure. Range of motion considers the quality of movement, end feel, and restricted or excessive range. Tenderness or pain is in an area or in specific tissues that may be provoked when palpated.

98. C: Planning is a stage that the client and the practitioner create with each other. In this stage, long-range treatment plans are made and are key to maintaining clients who receive treatments on a regular basis. The long-range treatment plans serve as a reminder for the client to take responsibility for his goal. It also gives both parties the opportunity to see the effectiveness of the treatment plan.

99. D: The main purposes for licenses and permits are to raise revenue and to protect the health and safety of the public. Before opening up a business, it is imperative to be aware of the local zoning requirements. This can be a difficult process because each locale has different zoning laws and it is not always clear which department issues the various permits necessary.

100. C: In a third-class lever system, a force is applied between the resistance and the fulcrum, where speed and distance traveled are increased at the expense of effective force. A third-class lever is the most common in the body; there are few first or second-class levers.

101. A: In Swedish massage, you should always massage towards the heart (centripetally). This means that movements should be directed upward along the lower parts of the body and limbs, and then downward from the head. This facilitates the flow of venous blood and lymph back toward the heart and other eliminatory organs.

102. D: Massage is safe during all trimesters as long as the pregnancy does not have any extenuating circumstances rendering it otherwise unsafe (such as symptoms of miscarriage or being classified as high risk). However, there are some techniques that should be avoided, such as deep connective tissue and myofascial release techniques, as well as putting sustained pressure in areas that are reflexology points associated with the uterus or ovaries.

103. A: Long reflexes are the most important in regulating visceral activities in most organs. Exceptions to this are the digestive tract and its associated glands; here, short reflexes provide most of the control and coordination needed for normal functions. All visceral reflexes are polysynaptic and are either long or short reflexes.

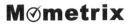

104. D: Kinetic energy is the energy of motion; it is energy that is doing work. Energy is the capacity to perform work, but movement or physical change cannot occur unless energy is provided. Kinetic energy is one of the two major types of energy that can cause movement or physical change; the other major type is potential energy.

105. A: Homeostasis is the internal balance of the body. The body strives to maintain this balance and is affected by any changes in the stresses that are posed by an external environment. These changes require the body to constantly compensate to maintain this delicate balance.

106. C: Psoriasis is a chronic inflammatory skin disorder where the skin renews itself every few days instead of every month. Since old skin cells do not slough off fast enough, they build up in thick patches. Psoriasis typically affects the scalp, elbows, knees, back, chest, and buttocks. Approximately 1-3% of the population has psoriasis and about 30% of people with it will develop arthritis.

107. B: The brain stem includes the mesencephalon, the pons, and the medulla oblongata. The mesencephalon is the midbrain, which contains nuclei that process visual and auditory information. The pons connects the cerebellum to the brain stem and contains nuclei involved with somatic and visceral motor control. The medulla oblongata relays sensory information to the thalamus and to other portions of the brain stem.

108. C: Countertransference occurs when the practitioner personalizes a therapeutic relationship by unconsciously projecting characteristics of someone from a former relationship onto a client. It often involves misperceptions and is usually subconscious but always detrimental to the therapeutic process. The opposite of this is called transference, which is what happens when a client negatively or positively personalizes a therapeutic relationship by subconsciously projecting characteristics of someone from a former relationship onto the massage practitioner.

109. D: The three most common learning styles among people are visual, auditory, and kinesthetic. Most people use all of these methods to process information, but one is usually dominant. People with visual learning styles tend to view the world in pictures and talk a little faster than average; people with auditory learning styles prefer to discuss things and are sensitive to noisy distractions; kinesthetic learners usually speak more slowly and like to touch items and experience sensations.

110. A: The capsular pattern refers to the proportional limitation of any joint this is controlled by muscular contractions. It is one of the concepts developed by Dr. James Cyriax that are invaluable when assessing range of motion. His system tests all of the joints to isolate lesions in the hard and soft tissues.

111. A: Massage can be indicated during and between gout attacks. Massage should be postponed if the client is experiencing fever or nausea during an attack period, but may be performed if those symptoms are not present as long as the affected joints are avoided. Massage is always indicated between attacks, unless other unrelated circumstances that result in contraindication are present.

112. C: The trigeminal nerve is the fifth cranial nerve. It is the largest cranial nerve and is classified as a mixed (motor and sensory) nerve. It is responsible for providing sensation to the face as well as supporting certain motor functions of the face and jaw, such as chewing. The trigeminal nerve branches into three parts: the ophthalmic nerve, the maxillary nerve, and the mandibular nerve.

113. D: All of the above. Common household disinfectants such as chlorine bleach are effective for disinfecting linens, implements, and surfaces. Ethyl is a type of alcohol that when used as a disinfectant, destroys most types of bacteria and viruses on surfaces. Cresol is another type of disinfectant that may be combined with other products to kill bacteria, viruses, and parasites.

114. C: Massage can reduce stress in cases of stable angina. It can also decrease the effects of the sympathetic nervous system, which holds partial responsibility for coronary artery constriction. However, it is important that clients have their necessary medications with them in the event of an angina attack during a treatment session.

115. A: Certain massage movements affect the blood and lymph channels in various ways. Along with increasing the permeability of the capillary beds, friction also hastens the flow of blood through superficial veins and increases the flow of interstitial fluid, which creates a healthier environment for cells.

116. C: The physiologic barrier is within the anatomic barrier and represents the comfortable end of soft tissue stretch during range of motion. It is the extent of easy movement allowed during passive or active movements. Along with restrictive barriers, it reflects conditions of bind and ease that is related to contractile muscle tissue and fascia.

117. A: A mechanical effect of friction is encouragement of phagocytosis due to the acceleration of circulation by aiding venous and lymph circulation. When friction is being used for this purpose, it should be applied alternately to the affected part and also to the tissues between it and the heart.

118. C: A dual relationship is any situation that combines the therapeutic relationship with a secondary relationship. The secondary relationship extends beyond the normal massage practitioner/client relationship. This may arise when someone the practitioner knows becomes a client, such as a family member, friend, work associate, or someone from the practitioner's church or other organization. It is also considered a dual relationship when services are being bartered.

119. A: It is better to pay monthly business statements with a business check because it provides better documentation than cash. It is also more ideal than using a personal check. It is acceptable to use a personal check occasionally; just post the expense under Petty Cash, note which account was used, then write a check to "petty cash" for the same amount to cash. It is best to create a separate identity for personal and financial reasons.

120. D: All of the choices listed are major contraindications to consider before administering massage. Normal body temperature ranges from 96.4°F to 99.1°F. Massage is not recommended when the temperature exceeds 99.4°F; massage would tend to work against the defense mechanisms of the body. Massaging a client with an acute infectious disease would intensify the illness as well as expose the therapist to the infection. Acute inflammation in a particular area is contraindicated because massage could further intensify the inflammation.

121. B: Gait is a pattern or manner of walking; it is similar to assessing posture but it takes place with the body in motion. Gait assessment is observing this manner. The client's gait should be viewed from the front, back, and both sides. It is done as the client does a relaxed walk for several times back and forth in front of the therapist.

122. C: Professional boundaries lay the foundation for an ethical practice. Respecting personal boundaries and maintaining professional boundaries ensures that the therapeutic relationship will be healthy for the client and will be void of ethical dilemmas. Boundaries can be professional, personal, physical, emotional, intellectual, and sexual; they are personal comfort zones that help maintain a sense of comfort and safety.

123. D: For a client with meningitis, massage should be postponed until the client has healed completely. Meningitis is usually caused by viruses or bacteria and is characterized by a severe headache, fever and chills, light sensitivity, a hyperextended stiff neck, and a red spotty rash. Vertigo, nausea, projectile vomiting, mental disorientation, and seizures may also occur as the condition progresses.

124. C: Gate control theory states that painful impulses are transmitted along small-diameter and large-diameter nerve fibers that run from nociceptors to the spinal cord and then to the brain. Stimulation of thermoreceptors or mechanoreceptors by rubbing, massaging, or icing is transmitted through the larger fibers, which suppress pain sensations at the gate where fibers enter the spinal column.

125. C: Serous glands secrete a watery solution that contains enzymes. An example of serous glands is the parotid salivary gland. Serous glands are a type of exocrine gland, along with mucous glands and mixed-exocrine glands. These exocrine glands are categorized by the types of secretions that they produce.

MBLEx Practice Test #3

1. Which circulatory structure is described as being responsible for the carrying of deoxygenated blood centripetally to the heart by way of valves to act against gravity?

    a. Arteries
    b. Veins
    c. Interstitial fluid
    d. Lymph

2. Which answer correctly names the three parts of the small intestine?

    a. Ilium, Ischium, pubis
    b. Ileum, Ischium, cecum
    c. Ileum, duodenum, cecum
    d. Ileum, duodenum, jejunum

3. The adrenal medulla is responsible for the conversion of amino acids into ____.

    a. T3 and T4.
    b. Epinephrine, norepinephrine, and dopamine.
    c. Aldosterone and testosterone.
    d. Oxytocin and vasopressin.

4. The most superficial layer of the epidermis is the ____.

    a. Stratum lucidum.
    b. Stratum corneum.
    c. Dermis.
    d. Stratum granulosum.

5. The following answer that is NOT associated with the lymphatic system is/are the ___.

    a. Spleen.
    b. Lymph nodes.
    c. Pituitary gland.
    d. Thymus gland.

6. The stationary end of a muscle is referred to as the _____.

    a. Insertion.
    b. Origin.
    c. Antagonist.
    d. Protagonist.

7. Which of the following describes the action of smooth muscle?

    a. Striated and voluntary
    b. Striated and involuntary
    c. Nonstriated and voluntary
    d. Nonstriated and involuntary

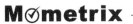

8. How many cranial nerves make up the peripheral nervous system?

    a. 12
    b. 11
    c. 13
    d. 15

9. The _____ is/are NOT a part of the nervous system.

    a. Brain
    b. Spinal cord
    c. Heart
    d. Sensory receptors

10. _____ is/are an automatic response used to diagnose nervous disorders and also to help maintain homeostasis.

    a. Reflexes
    b. Spasms
    c. Cramps
    d. Pain

11. The _____ plexus is responsible for nervous innervation to the upper extremities and certain neck and shoulder muscles.

    a. Lumbar
    b. Sacral
    c. Cervical
    d. Brachial

12. The two systems of the body that bring oxygen to the cells and eliminate carbon dioxide from the cells are the _____ and _____ systems.

    a. Respiratory and integumentary
    b. Circulatory and integumentary
    c. Respiratory and circulatory
    d. Circulatory and nervous

13. The _____ muscle is responsible for the act of inspiration and exhalation during normal breathing.

    a. Diaphragm
    b. External intercostals
    c. Internal intercostals
    d. Transversus abdominis

14. Which of the following is not part of the axial skeleton?

    a. Parietal bone
    b. Sternum
    c. Humerus
    d. Sacrum

15.___ are responsible for the eyes' black and white vision in dim light.

    a. Cones
    b. Rods
    c. Lens
    d. Corneas

16. What is the tubelike structure that carries urine from the kidney to the bladder?

    a. Ureter
    b. Glomerulus
    c. Islets of Langerhans
    d. Urethra

17. Which of the following does NOT describe a function of blood?

    a. Transports oxygen, carbon dioxide, nutrients, and waste
    b. Regulates pH, body temperature, and osmolarity
    c. Regulates hormones
    d. Creates clots and combats toxins

18. Which digestive hormone promotes secretion of gastric juices and is responsible for motility?

    a. Secretin
    b. Oxytocin
    c. Epinephrine
    d. Gastrin

19. The place at which bones meet is defined as a

    a. suture
    b. joint
    c. aponeurosis
    d. intersection

20. The main purpose of synovial fluid is to

    a. provide lubrication
    b. promote clotting
    c. promote muscle contraction
    d. excrete through the skin to maintain homeostasis

21. Flexing the elbow exhibits active movement for the following muscle:

    a. Triceps brachii
    b. Deltoid
    c. Latissimus dorsi
    d. Biceps brachii

22. How would passive range of motion (ROM) best be described?

    a. A client moves the requested part himself
    b. A client moves against the therapist at his request
    c. A client stays still
    d. A client's body part is moved by the therapist

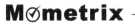

23. The following pathology is defined as fluid buildup from a lack of drainage in the lymph system:

    a. edema
    b. psoriasis
    c. dermatitis
    d. melanoma

24. What documentation is required to work inside a client's mouth?

    a. Signed history and release from the client
    b. Signed history and release from the client and verbal approval from the client
    c. Signed history and release from the client and verbal approval from his doctor
    d. Signed history and release from the client and written approval from her doctor

25. Which massage technique should be avoided when a client reports hypertension on their history form?

    a. Tapotement
    b. Centripetal strokes of any kind
    c. Centrifugal strokes of any kind
    d. Pressure touch

26. Pertaining to piriformis syndrome, which nerve is entrapped by the piriformis and other deep lateral rotators?

    a. Pudendal
    b. Sciatic
    c. Femoral
    d. Radial

27. When assessing a client complaining of chondromalacia patellae, the following group of muscles should be taken into consideration during treatment:

    a. Quadriceps
    b. Hamstrings
    c. Glutes
    d. Anterior compartment of the leg

28. Which of the following is NOT a cranial bone?

    a. Maxilla(e)
    b. Sphenoid
    c. Parietal
    d. Occipital

29. With what pathological condition is it absolutely contraindicated to perform massage therapy?

    a. History of a heart attack
    b. Active skin cancer
    c. Active deep tissue thrombosis
    d. Psoriasis

MBLEx Practice Test #3

30. Using light to moderate pressure with a rapid side-to-side motion is known as the technique of:

    a. Tapotement
    b. Pétrissage
    c. Pressure touch
    d. Vibration

31. When is it appropriate to begin visually assessing the client?

    a. As soon as the client walks in the door
    b. After the client has given their history
    c. After the client has gotten on the table
    d. Before the client has used the restroom

32. An individual muscle cell is called a(n):

    a. Leukocyte
    b. Adipocyte
    c. Myocyte
    d. Amino acid

33. The following occurs in the blood when heat is applied to the skin:

    a. Vasodilation
    b. Vasoconstriction
    c. Swelling
    d. Hypertension

34. Which of the following is NOT correct pertaining to the physiological effect that massage therapy has on muscles?

    a. Muscle tone is improved
    b. Muscle elasticity is improved
    c. Weak and tight muscle function is improved
    d. The temperature of the muscle is decreased by up to 1ºC.

35. Which of the following massage techniques is most commonly known for the movement of cellular waste from the muscles due to increased circulation?

    a. Pétrissage
    b. Effleurage
    c. Tapotement
    d. Touch

36. The following statement is true of the benefits of massage:

    a. The nervous system is stimulated
    b. The rate of breathing is decreased
    c. Trauma of any kind is decreased
    d. Decreases inflammation

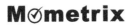

37. Which one of the following statements is *false* regarding the physiological effects of massage of the muscular system?

a. Increases healing time of strains
b. Decreases scar tissue
c. Increases range of motion
d. Reduces pain and swelling

38. Which is the correct classification for drugs defined as illegal, with no medical use, and a high potential for addictive behavior?

a. Schedule 1
b. Schedule 2
c. Schedule 3
d. Schedule 4

39. Which areas should a massage therapist not massage when a client reports a broken wrist?

a. Affected wrist and hand
b. Affected wrist only
c. Affected hand only
d. Affected forearm and wrist

40. Which of the following roots means "kidney?"

a. Nephro -
b. Pulmo -
c. Neuro -
d. Histo-

41. The term "endoscopy" means which of the following?

a. The use of a machine to obtain a live camera feed of the inside of the body
b. The use of a machine to obtain a live camera feed of the outside of the body
c. The use of an x-ray machine to obtain an image of the inside of the body
d. The use of a magnetic resonance imaging (MRI) machine to obtain a live feed of the outside of the body

42. Which one of the four signs listed below indicates an inflammatory response in the body?

a. Heat, redness, pain, swelling
b. Heat, pain, swelling, fever
c. Fever, swelling, hemorrhage, redness
d. Pain, swelling, fever, hemorrhage

43. During muscular contraction, the action potential is created by activating voltage-gated sodium channels down the axon toward the

a. Voltage-gated channels
b. Calcium channels
c. Neuromuscular junction
d. Acetylcholine receptors

44. Adenosine triphosphate (ATP) binds to which of the following during muscle contraction to release actin?

    a. Troponin
    b. Tropomyosin
    c. Actin
    d. Myosin

45. With regard to skeletal muscle, which of the following neurons travel from the muscle to the spinal cord during contraction?

    a. Motor neurons
    b. Muscle spindle cells
    c. Sensory neurons
    d. Golgi tendon organs

46. The rectus femoris' main actions are to

    a. Flex the hip and flex the knee
    b. Flex the hip and extend the knee
    c. Extend the hip and extend the knee
    d. Extend the hip and flex the knee

47. The insertion of the biceps brachii is located on the

    a. Ulnar tuberosity
    b. Humerus at the lateral supracondylar ridge
    c. Radial styloid process
    d. Radial tuberosity

48. The massage technique that can be used to increase heat production is called

    a. Kneading
    b. Stroking
    c. Vibration
    d. Stretching

49. Which of the following is a physiological effect that massage has on the integumentary system?

    a. Skin losing pallor
    b. Stimulation of sebaceous glands
    c. Decreased perspiration
    d. None of the above

50. Which one is NOT an example of an acute athletic injury?

    a. Dislocations
    b. Infections
    c. Contusions
    d. Sprains

51. Which actions does the elbow make when actively moving through the normal range of motion?

a. Adduction/abduction
b. Flexion/extension
c. Inversion/eversion
d. None of the above

52. A client complains of pain in his leg. He is unable to flex his knee. Which muscle or group of muscles is most likely affected?

a. Quadriceps
b. Gastrocnemius
c. Biceps brachii
d. Hamstrings

53. Which of the following is a contraindication for touch?

a. Numbness
b. Burns
c. Headache
d. None of these

54. Which of the following massage techniques is known to improve blood circulation and promote cellular waste movement?

a. Tapotement
b. Pressure touch
c. Friction
d. Reflex stroking

55. Friction would be contraindicated for which condition?

a. Edema
b. Sprains
c. Sciatica
d. Varicose veins

56. Centripetal friction should be performed in all of the following pathologies EXCEPT

a. Arthritis
b. Pain
c. Gout
d. Edema

57. Which of the following is NOT a contraindication for joint movement?

a. Synovitis
b. Fracture
c. Ankylosis
d. Rheumatoid arthritis

58. Joint pain can be relieved by all of the following EXCEPT

a. Pressure
b. Movements of the joint above
c. Massaging the area above the affected joint
d. Massaging the area below the affected joint

59. A client complains of anxiety from a recent stressful life event. Which stroke should not be used for the client's benefit?

a. Stroking
b. Pétrissage
c. Kneading
d. Percussion

60. Which of the following is NOT an absolute contraindication for massage?

a. Shock
b. Kidney failure
c. Hemorrhage
d. Arthritis

61. An indication for using cold hydrotherapy is

a. Cold hypersensitivity
b. Compromised superficial circulation
c. Strain
d. Heart attack

62. Which of the following is within the therapist's scope of practice to determine whether massage therapy is indicated for any client?

a. Taking a pulse/blood pressure
b. Checking his or her blood sugar
c. Performing an oral examination
d. All of the above

63. The kneading technique described as using the heel of the hand or the whole palmar surface is

a. Pétrissage
b. Digital
c. Palmar
d. Effleurage

64. To perform centripetal friction to the leg, the therapist would move

a. From the ankle to the patella
b. From the patella to the ankle
c. From the patella to the hip
d. From the hip to the patella

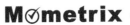

65. **Chucking is a useful massage technique to treat**

   a. Insomnia
   b. Headache
   c. Paralysis
   d. Tetanus

66. **Which of the following is not a form of percussion/tapotement?**

   a. Cupping
   b. Hacking
   c. Wringing
   d. Beating

67. **During the application of massage, which technique should be alternated with friction?**

   a. Wringing
   b. Joint movement
   c. Vibration
   d. Kneading

68. **When performing joint movement:**

   a. Stabilize the distal portion of the limb
   b. Move the proximal portion of the limb
   c. Shake the distal portion of the limb
   d. Stabilize the proximal portion of the limb

69. **The shifting of fluids from one part of the body to another is known as**

   a. Hydrophobia
   b. Osmosis
   c. Hydrostatic effect
   d. Hydrophilia

70. **Which of the following would provide the most stimulation?**

   a. Application of a heat pack
   b. Application of a cold pack
   c. A hot bath
   d. None of the above

71. **The acronym "RICE" means**

   a. Rest, ice, constrict, elevate
   b. Rest, ice, compression, exercise
   c. Rest, ice, compression, elevation
   d. Rest, ice, constrict, exercise

72. **Which of the following is an indication for heat therapy?**

   a. Strain
   b. Bleeding
   c. Contusion
   d. Fever

MBLEx Practice Test #3

73. **When applying cold to a client, which of the following is true?**
    a. It decreases metabolism
    b. It increases circulation
    c. It increases metabolism
    d. It decreases muscle tone

74. **The site where the muscle fiber and nerve fiber meet is known as the**
    a. Neurotransmitter
    b. Aponeurosis
    c. Joint
    d. Neuromuscular junction

75. **Which term best describes a sudden involuntary contraction of a muscle or group of muscles that does not cause pain?**
    a. Spasm
    b. Reflex
    c. Cramp
    d. Constriction

76. **Which of the following terms is also known as "muscle testing?"**
    a. Passive movement
    b. Active movement
    c. Assisted movement
    d. Resisted movement

77. **For support of the client, bolsters may be positioned under the client's ____ when prone and under the ____ when supine.**
    a. Ankles, knees
    b. Ankles, neck
    c. Ankles, lower back
    d. Hips, knees

78. **The appropriate temperature of a massage room is between**
    a. 60 and 66ºF
    b. 72 and 78ºF
    c. 75 and 80ºF
    d. 68 and 74ºF

79. **Which of the following may occur after a relaxation massage session?**
    a. Slight headache
    b. Bruising
    c. Decreased urine output
    d. Decreased appetite

80. **Which psychological pathology cannot be directly treated by massage therapy?**
    a. Depression
    b. Insomnia
    c. Anxiety
    d. Schizophrenia

214

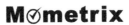

81. Which term is defined as the stage at which a therapeutic massage strategy is being determined and therapeutic modalities are selected?

    a. Performance
    b. Evaluation
    c. Planning
    d. Assessment

82. The purpose of a code of ethics is to

    a. Provide principles of correct and incorrect conduct
    b. Provide informed consent from a client
    c. Provide principles of good and evil
    d. Provide personal prejudices to place on the race and religion of clients

83. Which best describes how a therapist should follow ethical behavior?

    a. The therapist should conduct all actions and activities within the law
    b. The therapist should conduct all actions and activities within their best judgment
    c. The therapist should conduct all actions and activities within their scope of practice
    d. The therapist should conduct all actions and activities within their professional image

84. When is it ok to discuss a client's information with someone else?

    a. It is never ok to discuss a client's information with anyone
    b. It is ok to speak with the client's spouse and immediate family
    c. It is ok to speak with the client's friends
    d. It is always ok to discuss a client's information with anyone

85. How do ethics differ from laws?

    a. Ethics do not carry any punishment
    b. Laws do not carry any punishment
    c. Ethics may be punished in a variety of ways including fines, licensure revocation, and criminal trial
    d. Ethics violations are measured by degrees and can be punished by fines, probation, and community service

86. A professional boundary can be best described as

    a. The space of the client in a therapeutic relationship
    b. The space of the therapist in a therapeutic relationship
    c. The physical, emotional, and spiritual space between the client and therapist
    d. None of the above

87. In which of the following environments would it be the most difficult to maintain professional boundaries?

    a. The therapist's home
    b. The client's home
    c. The therapist's office
    d. The restroom

88. What word defines the personalization of a therapeutic relationship?
- a. Misconduct
- b. Countertransference
- c. Interpersonal communication
- d. None of the above

89. When a client asks the therapist out on a date in the massage session, what is the BEST way to handle the situation?
- a. The therapist should stop the massage and tell the client to leave
- b. The therapist should stop the massage and explain that if they were to go on a date, the therapist would have to first refer the client to another therapist and then they can begin a personal relationship
- c. The therapist should answer and then continue the massage
- d. The therapist should answer and then stop the massage

90. Which type of dual relationship is NOT acceptable?
- a. A therapist and client trade massages because the client is also a therapist
- b. A therapist and client are dating and have been engaging in sexual activity
- c. A therapist and client are business partners
- d. A therapist and client are friends and attend a spinning class together

91. Ethical behavior includes all of the following EXCEPT
- a. Legally acceptable behavior
- b. Boundaries
- c. Scope of practice
- d. Confidentiality

92. The study of morals, values, and principles is defined as
- a. Scope of practice
- b. Legal compliance
- c. Moral compliance
- d. Ethics

93. Which of the following is NOT out of the scope of practice for a therapist?
- a. Using electrical stimulation to excite/relax muscles
- b. Performing therapy inside the mouth with a prescription
- c. Telling a client to drink water
- d. Performing internal massage to the sacrococcygeal ligaments

94. When is it ok to tell a client to drink water?
- a. It is not ok; it is outside the scope of practice for a massage therapist
- b. It is ok after the treatment
- c. It is ok anytime
- d. It is ok only before the treatment

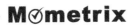

95. For a practitioner solely holding a massage therapy license, which of the following is the correct way to abbreviate their credentials?

   a. Dr. Jane Doe, LMT
   b. Mrs. Jane Doe, LMT
   c. Jane Doe, Ph.D., LMT
   d. Jane Doe, LMT, DO

96. Which of the following is NOT a personal hygiene guideline that should be practiced by a therapist?

   a. Brush teeth and use mouthwash when appropriate
   b. Keep hair fresh and styled appropriately so long hair does not touch the client
   c. Take time for relaxation and physical fitness
   d. Eat fast food when possible

97. Which of the following is the best definition of the word "virus"?

   a. Minute, unicellular microorganisms that have both plant and animal characteristics
   b. Parasitic microscopic agents that are capable of transmitting disease between organisms
   c. Eukaryotic microorganism that contains chitin in their cellular walls
   d. None of the above

98. Which of the following is considered the most effective safety practice to prevent the spread of disease?

   a. Showering
   b. Laundering sheets
   c. Washing hands
   d. Vacuuming

99. A substance that prevents infection by the killing of bacteria is known as a

   a. Disinfectant
   b. Sanitizer
   c. Sterilizer
   d. None of the above

100. What is the percentage of bleach solution used to clean up a spill of bodily fluids?

   a. 5%
   b. 10%
   c. 15%
   d. 20%

101. Where is the best place to store client records?

   a. File folder
   b. File folder inside of a box
   c. File folder inside of a locked box
   d. They can be placed anywhere

102. Having a home-based business has several advantages. Which is NOT an advantage?

a. No commute
b. Family members disrespecting boundaries
c. Be your own boss
d. Make your own schedule

103. Which of the following is a disadvantage of being self-employed?

a. Independence from employers
b. Do not have to worry about commission
c. Can have employees
d. Financial risk

104. What is the length of time that confidential client records are kept?

a. 1 year
b. 5 years
c. 8 years
d. 10 years

105. Outlining a business' purpose, setting goals, and stating an objective are known as

a. Financial planning
b. Presenting
c. Business planning
d. Accounting

106. Whose work was craniosacral therapy based on?

a. W. G. Sutherland
b. John Harvey Kellogg
c. Mark F. Beck
d. None of the above

107. Which of the following can be considered objective information?

a. Pain level assessment
b. Duration of pain
c. Client goals
d. Range of motion (ROM) testing

108. Where would the therapist document what the client has expressed?

a. Subjective
b. Objective
c. Assessment
d. Plan

109. Which of the following is NOT considered part of the endocrine system?

a. Thymus
b. Pancreas
c. Parathyroid
d. Pharynx

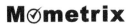

110. During an assessment, what is comparing one side of the body to the other known as?

    a. Unilateral symmetry
    b. Bilateral symmetry
    c. Balanced symmetry
    d. None of the above

111. Which of the following results of a muscle test should be referred to a doctor?

    a. Weak and painless muscle test
    b. No strength in the muscle
    c. Strong and painless muscle test
    d. Weak and painful muscle test

112. Assessing how the client walks and carries herself is known as

    a. Gait assessment
    b. Postural assessment
    c. Bilateral assessment
    d. Quadrilateral assessment

113. Which of the following conditions cannot be treated with massage?

    a. Tachycardia
    b. Atrophy of the heart muscle
    c. Myocarditis
    d. None of the above

114. Which of the following is the correct treatment order for carpal tunnel?

    a. Release muscles, increase range of motion (ROM), decrease pain
    b. Decrease pain, increase ROM, release muscles
    c. Increase ROM, decrease pain, release muscles
    d. Only the fascia should be worked

115. Why is it important to get a verbal intake?

    a. The client may have forgotten to write something on their form
    b. It is faster than a written intake
    c. It takes less time
    d. None of the above

116. Which of the following is NOT a massage therapy modality?

    a. Reiki
    b. Jiu-jitsu
    c. Thai
    d. Polarity therapy

117. A client complains of numbness and tingling down her left arm. What should the beginning treatment plan include?

    a. Left neck, shoulder, arm, and wrist
    b. Left neck
    c. Left neck and shoulder
    d. Left neck and arm

118. During a massage, the therapist feels a warm and red raised area on the client's arm. There is no wound, but the client expresses that it is painful. What is this area most likely?

a. Tumor
b. Infection
c. Inflammation
d. Contusion

119. What is the belly of a muscle referred to in the Shiatsu method of massage therapy?

a. Hiro
b. Hara
c. Hilot
d. None of the above

120. Which client position is best for on-site corporate massage events?

a. Prone
b. Supine
c. Seated
d. Standing

121. Which method of massage therapy was developed by Boris Chaitow and Stanley Leif to relieve compressed nerves that refer pain to other parts of the body?

a. Polarity therapy
b. Reiki
c. Neuromuscular therapy
d. Shiatsu

122. The focus of applied kinesiology is

a. Strengthen and tone muscle tissue
b. Emotional release
c. Increasing structural balance and functionality
d. Meditation and relaxation

123. During a relaxation massage session, a client is expressing that his pain is unbearable. What is the best course of action?

a. Ignore him
b. Tell him to relax
c. Ease off the pressure, and ask him if his pain has decreased
d. Tell him it is part of the massage

124. When checking range of motion (ROM) on a client, the therapist notices limited extension in her knee. Which muscle(s) should be addressed?

a. Quadriceps
b. Hamstrings
c. Adductors
d. Glutes

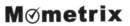

125. Upon bilaterally comparing the client's calves, one side is much more firm than the other. This can be due to all of the following EXCEPT

    a. Hypertonicity
    b. Overuse
    c. Postural/gait Imbalance
    d. Nerve damage

Answer Key and Explanations for Test #3

1. B: The answer arteries is incorrect because they are the structure responsible for carrying blood away from the heart. Interstitial fluid is incorrect because it is the fluid between cells and tissues, not responsible for moving at all. Lymph is incorrect because it is made up of the white blood cells and immune cells. It is not a structure that is used to move blood.

2. D: Ilium, Ischium, pubis are incorrect because these are the bones of the pelvis. Ileum, Ischium, cecum are incorrect because the ischium is part of the pelvis, and the cecum is part of the large intestine. Ileum, duodenum, cecum are incorrect because the cecum is part of the large intestine.

3. B: T3 and T4 are incorrect because these hormones are made in the thyroid gland. Aldosterone and testosterone are incorrect because the adrenal cortex and testosterone is produced in the gonads. Oxytocin and vasopressin are incorrect because these hormones are made in the pituitary gland.

4. B: The stratum lucidum is incorrect because this is the layer only present in the thick skin of the fingers and the soles of the feet. Dermis is incorrect because the dermis is the layer of skin containing collagen and elastic fibers. Stratum granulosum is incorrect because this is the middle layer of the epidermis.

5. C: Spleen is incorrect because the spleen is the largest lymph tissue in the body responsible for phagocytosis. Lymph nodes are incorrect because the lymph nodes are part of the lymph system and hold lymph in places throughout the body. The thymus gland is incorrect because it is part of the lymph system because it provides the site for the maturation of T cells.

6. B: Insertion is incorrect because it is the moving end of a muscle. Antagonist is incorrect because the antagonist is a muscle that performs the opposite action to another muscle. Protagonist is incorrect because the antagonist is a muscle that performs a similar action to another muscle.

7. D: Striated and voluntary are incorrect because they describe skeletal muscle. Striated and involuntary are incorrect because they do not describe any muscle fibers of the body. Nonstriated and voluntary are incorrect because they do not describe any muscle fibers of the body.

8. A: There are 12 cranial nerves: olfactory, optic, oculomotor, trochlear, trigeminal, abducens, facial, vestibulocochlear, glossopharyngeal, vagus, spinal accessory, and hypoglossal.

9. C: The brain, spinal cord, and sensory receptors are incorrect because they are part of the nervous system.

10. A: Spasms are not correct because spasms do not assist with maintaining homeostasis, nor are they solely used to diagnose nervous disorders. Cramps are not correct because cramps do not assist with maintaining homeostasis, nor are they solely used to diagnose nervous disorders. Pain is not correct because pain does not assist with maintaining homeostasis, nor is it solely used to diagnose nervous disorders.

11. D: Lumbar is incorrect because the lumbar plexus innervates the legs, genitals, and parts of the abdomen. Sacral is incorrect because the sacral plexus innervates the glutes, perineum, and parts of the legs. Cervical is incorrect because the cervical plexus innervates the skin and muscles of the head and neck, cranial nerves, and diaphragm.

222

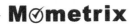

12. C: Respiratory and integumentary is incorrect because the integumentary system is not responsible for any type of cellular respiration. Circulatory and integumentary is incorrect because the integumentary system is not responsible for any type of respiration. Circulatory and nervous is incorrect because the nervous system is not responsible for any type of respiration.

13. A: External intercostals are incorrect because the external intercostals' action is to push air out of the lungs during abnormal breathing, like breathing deeply. Internal intercostals are incorrect because the internal intercostals' action is to assist the diaphragm by pulling air into the lungs during deep breathing. Transversus abdominis is incorrect because this muscle's action is to compress the abdomen.

14. C: Parietal bone is incorrect because this skull bone is part of the axial skeleton. Sternum is incorrect because the sternum and ribs are part of the axial skeleton. Sacrum is incorrect because this bone is part of the axial skeleton, along with the other vertebrae.

15. B: Cones are incorrect because cones are responsible for seeing color and visual acuity. Lens is incorrect because this anatomical structure focuses the light for clear vision. Corneas are incorrect because these anatomical structures refract light.

16. A: Glomerulus is incorrect because this is a functional structure of the kidney. Islets of Langerhans are incorrect because this is a functional structure of the kidney. Urethra is incorrect because this is the tube structure from the bladder to the external body that carries urine for elimination.

17. C: Regulates hormones — this is correct because the blood does not regulate hormones; this is the function of the endocrine system. Transports oxygen, carbon dioxide, nutrients, and waste is incorrect: this is a function of blood. Regulates pH, body temperature, and osmolarity is incorrect, this is a function of blood. Creates clots and combats toxins are incorrect, these are a function of blood.

18. D: Secretin is incorrect because secreting promotes the secretion of bicarbonate. Oxytocin is incorrect because oxytocin plays a role in childbirth. Epinephrine is incorrect because epinephrine is released during times of stress.

19. B: Suture is not correct because a suture is a "stitch" of bone. Aponeurosis is not correct because this is a layer of tendons. Intersection is not correct because it is not an anatomical term.

20. A: Synovial fluid is only used to lubricate joints and to reduce the amount of friction between moving bones. It does not promote clotting, which is part of the circulatory system. Muscle contraction is performed by myocytes, and sebaceous glands are responsible for excretions through the skin.

21. D: The triceps brachii extend the elbow. The deltoid does not attach at the elbow; it moves the shoulder. The latissimus dorsi also does not attach at the elbow; it moves the arm.

22. D: Active movement is when a client moves the part on their own. Resistive movement is when the client moves against the therapist, and no movement is made when the client stays still.

23. A: Psoriasis is a skin disorder due to skin cells dying too rapidly. Dermatitis is an inflammation of the skin. Melanoma is a type of skin cancer.

24. D: It is mandatory to obtain not only a prescription from the client's doctor for inside her mouth because without this document, it is outside the scope of practice for a therapist to perform massage inside the mouth. It is also mandatory for a therapist to obtain a written history and release from the client prior to any therapeutic treatment.

25. B: Centripetal strokes should be avoided because the strokes are made toward the heart, increasing blood pressure and stressing the client's circulatory system.

26. B: The sciatic nerve runs between the body of the piriformis and the gluteus muscles. The pudendal nerve is just lateral to the sacrum, but it is not associated with piriformis syndrome. The femoral and radial nerves are located in the leg and arm, respectively.

27. A: The quadriceps should be addressed because the patella is encased in the tendon of the quads. This would be most beneficial because releasing and stretching the quadriceps would provide the most benefit regarding pain and range of motion compared to the hamstrings, glutes, and anterior compartment of the leg.

28. A: Maxilla(e) is correct because the sphenoid, parietal, and occipital bones are cranial bones.

29. C: Massage therapy is absolutely contraindicated in patients with a deep vein thrombosis (DVT). A DVT is a large clot in a vein, most often found in the leg. If massaged, the clot may loosen and/or break apart creating what is called an embolus. An embolus is a portion of a clot that moves through the vascular system and can lodge in the heart, lungs, or brain and cause severe, even deadly, complications. Individuals with a known DVT should not receive a massage. Individuals with a history of a heart attack or active skin cancer can be massaged using careful consideration with regard to techniques, as well as written consent from their doctor. Psoriasis is not contraindicated, unless the patient experiences pain or has open sores.

30. D: Tapotement is a type of percussion, with the hands repetitively striking the skin. Pétrissage is a kneading motion. Pressure touch is the placement of the hands with light pressure on the skin.

31. A: It is appropriate to assess the client as soon as they walk in the door because the therapist can gauge their natural gait, posture, and any other indications of neuromuscular imbalance.

32. C: A leukocyte is a white blood cell. An adipocyte is a fat cell. An amino acid is a building block of proteins, and it is a collection of organic atoms bonded together.

33. A: Vasoconstriction is caused when cold is applied to the skin. Swelling can be possible when heat is applied, but it is not directly correlated with heat application. It is also a cause of vasodilation. Hypertension is a slight effect of when cold is applied to the skin.

34. A: During massage, the myocytes are never enlarged. Blood can flow through the muscle more easily, but the tone of the muscle is not affected.

35. A: Effleurage, tapotement, and touch do not have an effect on circulation.

36. B: The nervous system can be stimulated or repressed, trauma is usually decreased, and inflammation may or may not be affected by massage.

37. A: Massage decreases the healing time of strains, decreases scar tissue, increases range of motion, and reduces pain and swelling.

38. A: Schedule 1 drugs are classified as illegal, and all the other schedule drugs are not.

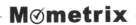

39. A: It is important to only work on the part proximal to the injured part because manipulating the part below can be painful for the client, or this can cause longer healing times.

40. A: Pulmo- means lung, neuro- means nerve, and histo- means liver.

41. A: Endo- means inside and -scopy means scope.

42. A: Pain, fever, and hemorrhage are not always present with inflammation.

43. C: The neuromuscular junction is where nerves meet muscle and where the action potential is carried for contraction. Mitochondria are the energy powerhouses of cells. Calcium channels play a part in action potentials, but they do not receive the action potential. Acetylcholine receptors receive acetylcholine, but not action potentials.

44. D: Troponin is attached to the protein tropomyosin during muscle contraction. Actin and myosin slide past each other during muscle contraction.

45. C: Motor neurons run from the spinal cord to the skeletal muscle to control voluntary muscle contraction. Muscle spindle cells are sensory receptors in the belly of a muscle. Golgi tendon organs are sensory receptors in the tendon to detect when and how much a muscle is being stretched.

46. B: The rectus femoris originates at the anterior inferior iliac spine and inserts at the aponeurosis in the patella. The muscle covers two joints; it flexes the hip and extends the knee.

47. D: The biceps brachii inserts at the bicipital aponeurosis and the radial tuberosity.

48. A: Kneading is correct because the muscle is picked up off of the muscle, manipulated, and placed back again on the muscle. Stroking does not create any heat because it is simply a nervous stimulation of the superficial skin. Stretching does not create any heat when the muscles are stretched. Vibration creates some heat due to the muscle being manipulated laterally, but it does not create any significant amount of heat.

49. B: Skin losing pallor and decreased perspiration are not physiological effects of massage on the integumentary system. Skin reddening and increased perspiration, as well as stimulation of the sebaceous glands are a few physiological effects of massage on the integumentary system.

50. B: Infections are not an acute athletic injury because there is not one specific incident that causes an infection that can be determined as the trauma. An infection takes time to develop, but dislocations, contusions, and sprains do not.

51. B: The elbow is a hinge joint and only has two actions — flexion and extension.

52. D: The hamstrings are responsible for flexing the knee and extending the hip. The quadriceps flexes the hip and extends the knee. The biceps brachii flexes the forearm and supinates the arm. The gastrocnemius contributes to the plantarflexion of the ankle.

53. B: Burns are a contraindication for touch because they are extremely sensitive to touch. Touching a client with burns can cause pain and cause increased healing time for the patient.

54. C: Friction is specifically known to move blood more quickly through the body by generating heat and increasing circulation which in turn promotes cellular waste movement. This effect is even employed to help neonatal infants with jaundice as increased circulation helps the kidneys to remove the excess bilirubin from the blood.

55. D: Friction is contraindicated for varicose veins because the veins are no longer properly working, and friction can increase the amount of varicose veins that a client has. Friction is beneficial for edema to drain fluid. Friction can decrease the healing time of strains, and it can improve blood flow to the muscles in the lumbar spine to treat sciatica.

56. C: Gout is the buildup of uric acid in the joints, and when centripetal friction is used, this can cause the uric acid to move to other joints and worsen the condition. Arthritis, pain, and edema will lessen with friction due to the improvement in circulation and elimination of cellular waste from the tissues.

57. D: Joint movement for rheumatoid arthritis (RA) is beneficial because it can increase the synovial fluid around the joint and bring nutrients to it, decreasing inflammation. Synovitis, fractures, and ankylosis are all immobilizing conditions, and the joints in, on, or around them should not be moved to reduce the risk of increased pain and healing time.

58. D: Massaging the area below the affected joint would not be beneficial because the area above may be manipulated inadvertently so that the pain in the joint above is increased.

59. D: Percussion is a stimulating technique to the nerves of the body, while stroking, pétrissage, and kneading are all sedative. Any type of neurological disorder derived from stress should use sedative techniques during treatment.

60. D: Arthritis is not a contraindication for massage because joint movement and other techniques are beneficial to reducing the inflammation of arthritis. Shock, kidney failure, and hemorrhage all add a risk of death to the client if he or she is massaged during acute and even chronic phases of these pathologies due to the fluctuation in blood pressure, increase in circulation, and cellular waste in the bloodstream.

61. C: A strain can be treated with cold hydrotherapy because of the vasoconstrictive properties that can reduce inflammation. Cold hydrotherapy should not be used in cases of cold hypersensitivity, compromised superficial circulation, or heart attack because these pathologies would worsen immediately or cause a delayed response, worsening the condition.

62. A: Taking a pulse/blood pressure is correct because the other three procedures are out of the scope of practice of a massage therapist.

63. C: Palmar kneading uses the palm of the hand, pétrissage and effleurage use the whole hand, and digital kneading uses only the fingers to perform the technique.

64. A: "Centripetal" means toward the heart or from inferior to superior in most cases.

65. D: Tetanus is the rigidity of a muscle. Chucking is useful to "reset" the muscle spindle cells to allow the muscle to relax. Cupping, hacking, and beating are percussive movements that may cause the muscle to tense up more.

66. C: Wringing is a type of kneading. Cupping, hacking, and beating are all forms of percussion.

67. D: Friction should always be alternated with kneading to promote the movement of cellular waste out of the body.

68. D: If the proximal portion of the limb is not stabilized, stress will be placed on any joints proximal to the joint that the therapist is working on, possibly causing pain. This will also inhibit joint movement.

69. B: Hydrophobia is the fear of water, and hydrophilia is the love of water. Osmosis is the movement of cellular molecules in a solvent from an area of lower concentration to a higher concentration.

70. B: Cold hydrotherapy is generally stimulative, and heat is generally sedative. To remember this, think of how you feel in a cold shower versus a warm shower.

71. C: Rest means to rest the injured part by keeping it immobile as much as possible. Ice means to ice it regularly to reduce inflammation and promote healing. Compression means to wrap or bandage the area to prevent infection or bruising. Elevation means to keep the injured part at or above the heart to promote draining of inflammation and cellular waste.

72. A: Bleeding, contusion, and fever are all contraindications for heat therapy because they can worsen with heat. Strains are indicated for heat because the heat vasodilates the blood vessels and allows for freshly oxygenated blood to rush in and promote healing.

73. A: Cold decreases the metabolism due to vasoconstriction. Heat therapy increases circulation and metabolism. Exercise increases muscle tone.

74. D: A neurotransmitter is a form of communication between nerves, an aponeurosis is where several tendons meet, and a joint is where two bones meet.

75. A: A reflex is a sudden movement of a muscle due to outside stimulation. A cramp is like a spasm, but the client feels pain as well. Constriction is not a medical term for any condition.

76. D: Passive movement is when the therapist moves the body part for the client. Active movement is when the client moves the body part for the therapist. Assisted movement is when both the therapist and the client move the body part together.

77. A: The client should have any joints that flex toward the table supported when supine, as well as prone. Some clients also prefer their neck supported when supine for this reason.

78. B: According to the Ohio State Medical Board and the *American Massage Therapy Association (AMTA)* ethics, the room temperature should be between 72 and 78ºF.

79. A: During any massage session, the client should not have any bruising. The client may have a slight headache, increased urine output due to the cellular waste in the bloodstream, and increased appetite due to massage therapy's sedative properties that activate a client's parasympathetic nervous system.

80. D: Schizophrenia cannot be directly treated by massage because it is a psychological condition that cannot be treated by activating the client's parasympathetic nervous system, as can be done with depression, insomnia, and anxiety.

81. C: Planning is also the P in SOAP notes. Assessment is determining which pathological and neuromuscular conditions are present. Evaluation can be categorized as taking a history and learning subjectively and objectively about the client. Performance is not a part of massage therapy's strategies.

82. A: Although informed consent and principles of good and evil can be considered a part of ethics, it is not the purpose of ethics. Personal prejudices are considered unethical.

83. C: It is very important that the therapist put their scope of practice first as their guidelines for all behavior. Because ethics are always lawful, the therapist will most always be following the law. Unfortunately, a therapist's best judgment and professional image are not always ethical, and they should not be considered when following ethical behavior.

84. A: It is both unethical and a violation of HIPAA to discuss a client's information with anyone but the client.

85. C: Although laws are harsh, ethical issues are often more detrimental because they can tarnish a therapist's reputation and cause other difficulties. Laws do not take ethics into consideration and usually only have monetary or time-serving-type penalties.

86. C: A professional boundary includes not only the space of the client and therapist, but the emotional and spiritual space as well. A client can violate one boundary without violating the others.

87. B: The client's home is the most difficult environment in which to maintain professional boundaries because the client's home is usually more of an informal environment and the client has the "power" to direct the session how they'd like to if the therapist does not exhibit himself as a professional practicing within his scope.

88. B: Misconduct is the unethical behavior of a therapist. Interpersonal communication is the written, verbal, or otherwise means of conveying a message to another.

89. B: A therapist should NEVER start a dual relationship in session and should always communicate with the client as clearly and nicely as possible, while making sure that the client understands. It is also imperative to explain the scope of practice and to convey oneself as an ethical professional.

90. B: This is an example of a dual relationship that is unethical due to the absence of boundaries between client and therapist.

91. A: Legally acceptable behavior is not always concurrent with ethical behavior. In the eye of the law, a therapist can break a law while acting ethically: Some may argue that Dr. Kevorkian, who assisted patients with committing suicide, was acting ethically, but he also broke the law by being an accomplice to murder.

92. D: Scope of practice is a set of rules drawn out to clearly define what a medical professional can and cannot do. Legal compliance is simply following laws. Moral compliance is simply following one's own morals.

93. B: Telling a client to drink water is out of the scope of practice because this is telling a client what to do in terms of ingestion. Internal massage is not in the scope of practice, except in the mouth with a written prescription from a doctor. Electrical stimulation is only in the scope of practice of chiropractors and physical therapists.

94. A: Telling a client to drink water is out of the scope of practice because this is telling a client what to do in terms of ingestion.

95. B: Jane Doe does not have any other medical license or credentials, so it is never appropriate to put Dr., Ph.D., or DO anywhere in her name.

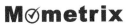

96. D: A therapist's diet is their choice, but it is not a hygienic guideline to eat fast food when possible.

97. B: Answer A describes bacteria, and answer C describes a fungus.

98. C: Although showering, laundering sheets, and vacuuming are good safety practices, hand washing is proven to be the number one way to prevent the spread of germs.

99. A: A sanitizer kills germs and bacteria but not all bacteria. A sterilizer is also a cleaner, but it is more widely used to kill bacteria on surfaces.

100. B: According to the State Medical Board of Ohio and the Federation of State Medical Boards (FSMB), the correct percentage solution is 10%.

101. C: According to the Federation of State Medical Boards (FSMB), all confidential client information should be organized in a locked box or filing cabinet.

102. B: No commute, being one's own boss, and making one's own schedule are great advantages of a home business. Family members not respecting boundaries is one of the drawbacks of this setup.

103. D: Independence from employers, no longer worrying about commission, and the possibility of having employees are great advantages of being self-employed, but there is a high level of financial risk involved.

104. D: Per the Federation of State Medical Boards (FSMB), the minimum amount of time a therapist should keep their confidential client records is 10 years.

105. C: Financial planning, presenting, and accounting are all subsets of business planning.

106. A: John Kellogg invented massage therapy; Mark Beck is an author who worked from Kellogg's massage information.

107. D: Range of motion (ROM) testing is objective because it is information that is observed by the therapist. Pain level assessments, duration of pain, and client goals are subjective because only the client can determine this information.

108. A: Subjective is what the "subject" has told the therapist. Objective is what "objects" the therapist has found. Assessment is the determination of pathologies and neuromuscular conditions, and plan is a treatment strategy for the session.

109. D: The thymus, pancreas, and parathyroid are all parts of the endocrine system, whereas the pharynx is part of the respiratory system.

110. B: Bilateral means both sides, and symmetry is defined as similarity from one side to the other. Unilateral means one side, and balanced symmetry does not allude to comparing one side of the body to the other.

111. D: A weak and painful muscle test could describe a serious sprain or strain that may need to be operated on, or it is a symptom of a neurological issue. A weak and painless muscle test arises from atrophy. A strong and painless muscle test is normal, and no strength in the muscle can also be from atrophy.

112. A: Postural assessment is more likely to describe when a client is standing still. A bilateral assessment is comparing each side of the body against the other. Quadrilateral assessment is not a term used in massage therapy.

113. C: Myocarditis is not treatable with massage therapy because the heart cannot directly or indirectly be treated to reduce the inflammation of the pericardial sac. Tachycardia can be treated with any centrifugal and/or sedative techniques. Atrophy of the heart muscle can be treated with several sessions of light centripetal strokes.

114. A: It is important to first release any hypertensive muscles to make way for effective stretching to then increase range of motion. Pain should always be last on a therapist's task list because pain is subjective and just because a client feels less pain does not mean that a muscle has been released or that the functionality of the area has increased.

115. A: It is always important to discuss the massage therapy session and review the client's history before beginning treatment, because the client almost always has a more elaborate explanation regarding their goals. This always gives the therapist the opportunity to ask questions and get more specific information not obtainable on a brief history form.

116. B: Reiki, Thai massage, and polarity therapy are all common modalities in massage therapists are trained. Jiu-jitsu is a Brazilian martial art.

117. A: It is important to treat the client's entire left upper extremity, including the neck, because it may be difficult to determine where the nerve impingement is originating.

118. C: The four signs of inflammation are redness, swelling, heat, and pain.

119. B: Hara is the belly of a muscle in Shiatsu massage.

120. C: Because corporate massage events are most often held in offices, it is best for the clients to be seated, due to the professional atmosphere and lack of time that the clients may have. They also do not have to be concerned about disrobing.

121. C: Reiki was developed by Usui in Japan in the early 1900s. Polarity therapy was developed by Randolph Stone, D.O., D.C., N.D. Shiatsu was developed by the Japanese before early civilization.

122. C: The focus of exercise is to strengthen and tone muscle tissue. The purpose of Touch for Health and other energy therapies is for emotional release. A variety of therapies, not including applied kinesiology, have a focus on meditation and relaxation.

123. C: It is important to be in communication with the client and to make him feel as comfortable as possible. Ignoring him will not build trust and is rude. Telling the client to relax is to not reciprocate the communication between client and therapist, and it can also prevent a trusting professional relationship. Telling him it is part of the massage is also inconsiderate and will not build trust.

124. A: The quadriceps are the group of muscles that extend the knee, and during a range of motion test, they can be responsible for limited extension of the knee.

125. D: Nerve damage does not change the size of a muscle with regard to bilateral comparison. Hypertonicity, overuse, and postural/gait imbalance are all possible outcomes of one side exhibiting a firmer touch.

Image Credits

Muscles That Assist in the Respiratory Process "The Diaphragm" by Openstax Anatomy & Physiology Chapter 11.4 (https://cnx.org/contents/FPtK1zmh@15.2:b3YG6PIp@10/11-4-Axial-Muscles-of-the-Abdominal-Wall-and-Thorax)

Spine Muscles: "Muscles of the Posterior Neck and the Back" by Openstax Anatomy & Physiology Chapter 11.3 (https://cnx.org/contents/FPtK1zmh@15.2:_xq2eUyd@9/11-3-Axial-Muscles-of-the-Head-Neck-and-Back)

Mastication Muscles: "Muscles That Move the Lower Jaw" by Openstax Anatomy & Physiology Chapter 11.3 (https://cnx.org/contents/FPtK1zmh@15.2:_xq2eUyd@9/11-3-Axial-Muscles-of-the-Head-Neck-and-Back)

Eye Muscles: "Muscles That Move the Eyes" by Openstax Anatomy & Physiology Chapter 11.3 (https://cnx.org/contents/FPtK1zmh@15.2:_xq2eUyd@9/11-3-Axial-Muscles-of-the-Head-Neck-and-Back)

Facial Expression Muscles: "Muscles That Create Facial Expression" by Openstax Anatomy & Physiology Chapter 11.3 (https://cnx.org/contents/FPtK1zmh@15.2:_xq2eUyd@9/11-3-Axial-Muscles-of-the-Head-Neck-and-Back)

Synovial Joint: "Synovial Joints" by Openstax Anatomy & Physiology Chapter 9.4 (https://cnx.org/contents/FPtK1zmh@15.2:bFtYymxt@8/9-4-Synovial-Joints)

Types of Synovial Joints: "Types of Synovial Joints" by Openstax Anatomy & Physiology Chapter 9.4 (https://cnx.org/contents/FPtK1zmh@15.2:bFtYymxt@8/9-4-Synovial-Joints)

Varicose Veins: "Varicose veins affecting the lower leg" by Welcome Images (https://commons.wikimedia.org/wiki/File:Varicose_veins_affecting_the_lower_leg_Wellcome_L0061800.jpg)

Anatomic Position: "Anatomical Position" by Openstax Anatomical Terms (https://cnx.org/contents/Gko70fNo@1/Anatomical-Terms)

LICENSED UNDER CC BY-SA 3.0 (CREATIVECOMMONS.ORG/LICENSES/BY-SA/3.0/DEED.EN)

Planes of Movement: "Human anatomy planes" by YassineMrabet (https://commons.wikimedia.org/wiki/File:Human_anatomy_planes.svg)

How to Overcome Test Anxiety

Just the thought of taking a test is enough to make most people a little nervous. A test is an important event that can have a long-term impact on your future, so it's important to take it seriously and it's natural to feel anxious about performing well. But just because anxiety is normal, that doesn't mean that it's helpful in test taking, or that you should simply accept it as part of your life. Anxiety can have a variety of effects. These effects can be mild, like making you feel slightly nervous, or severe, like blocking your ability to focus or remember even a simple detail.

If you experience test anxiety—whether severe or mild—it's important to know how to beat it. To discover this, first you need to understand what causes test anxiety.

Causes of Test Anxiety

While we often think of anxiety as an uncontrollable emotional state, it can actually be caused by simple, practical things. One of the most common causes of test anxiety is that a person does not feel adequately prepared for their test. This feeling can be the result of many different issues such as poor study habits or lack of organization, but the most common culprit is time management. Starting to study too late, failing to organize your study time to cover all of the material, or being distracted while you study will mean that you're not well prepared for the test. This may lead to cramming the night before, which will cause you to be physically and mentally exhausted for the test. Poor time management also contributes to feelings of stress, fear, and hopelessness as you realize you are not well prepared but don't know what to do about it.

Other times, test anxiety is not related to your preparation for the test but comes from unresolved fear. This may be a past failure on a test, or poor performance on tests in general. It may come from comparing yourself to others who seem to be performing better or from the stress of living up to expectations. Anxiety may be driven by fears of the future—how failure on this test would affect your educational and career goals. These fears are often completely irrational, but they can still negatively impact your test performance.

Elements of Test Anxiety

As mentioned earlier, test anxiety is considered to be an emotional state, but it has physical and mental components as well. Sometimes you may not even realize that you are suffering from test anxiety until you notice the physical symptoms. These can include trembling hands, rapid heartbeat, sweating, nausea, and tense muscles. Extreme anxiety may lead to fainting or vomiting. Obviously, any of these symptoms can have a negative impact on testing. It is important to recognize them as soon as they begin to occur so that you can address the problem before it damages your performance.

The mental components of test anxiety include trouble focusing and inability to remember learned information. During a test, your mind is on high alert, which can help you recall information and stay focused for an extended period of time. However, anxiety interferes with your mind's natural processes, causing you to blank out, even on the questions you know well. The strain of testing during anxiety makes it difficult to stay focused, especially on a test that may take several hours. Extreme anxiety can take a huge mental toll, making it difficult not only to recall test information but even to understand the test questions or pull your thoughts together.

Effects of Test Anxiety

Test anxiety is like a disease—if left untreated, it will get progressively worse. Anxiety leads to poor performance, and this reinforces the feelings of fear and failure, which in turn lead to poor performances on subsequent tests. It can grow from a mild nervousness to a crippling condition. If allowed to progress, test anxiety can have a big impact on your schooling, and consequently on your future.

Test anxiety can spread to other parts of your life. Anxiety on tests can become anxiety in any stressful situation, and blanking on a test can turn into panicking in a job situation. But fortunately, you don't have to let anxiety rule your testing and determine your grades. There are a number of relatively simple steps you can take to move past anxiety and function normally on a test and in the rest of life.

Physical Steps for Beating Test Anxiety

While test anxiety is a serious problem, the good news is that it can be overcome. It doesn't have to control your ability to think and remember information. While it may take time, you can begin taking steps today to beat anxiety.

Just as your first hint that you may be struggling with anxiety comes from the physical symptoms, the first step to treating it is also physical. Rest is crucial for having a clear, strong mind. If you are tired, it is much easier to give in to anxiety. But if you establish good sleep habits, your body and mind will be ready to perform optimally, without the strain of exhaustion. Additionally, sleeping well helps you to retain information better, so you're more likely to recall the answers when you see the test questions.

Getting good sleep means more than going to bed on time. It's important to allow your brain time to relax. Take study breaks from time to time so it doesn't get overworked, and don't study right before bed. Take time to rest your mind before trying to rest your body, or you may find it difficult to fall asleep.

Along with sleep, other aspects of physical health are important in preparing for a test. Good nutrition is vital for good brain function. Sugary foods and drinks may give a burst of energy but this burst is followed by a crash, both physically and emotionally. Instead, fuel your body with protein and vitamin-rich foods.

Also, drink plenty of water. Dehydration can lead to headaches and exhaustion, especially if your brain is already under stress from the rigors of the test. Particularly if your test is a long one, drink water during the breaks. And if possible, take an energy-boosting snack to eat between sections.

Along with sleep and diet, a third important part of physical health is exercise. Maintaining a steady workout schedule is helpful, but even taking 5-minute study breaks to walk can help get your blood pumping faster and clear your head. Exercise also releases endorphins, which contribute to a positive feeling and can help combat test anxiety.

When you nurture your physical health, you are also contributing to your mental health. If your body is healthy, your mind is much more likely to be healthy as well. So take time to rest, nourish your body with healthy food and water, and get moving as much as possible. Taking these physical steps will make you stronger and more able to take the mental steps necessary to overcome test anxiety.

Mental Steps for Beating Test Anxiety

Working on the mental side of test anxiety can be more challenging, but as with the physical side, there are clear steps you can take to overcome it. As mentioned earlier, test anxiety often stems from lack of preparation, so the obvious solution is to prepare for the test. Effective studying may be the most important weapon you have for beating test anxiety, but you can and should employ several other mental tools to combat fear.

First, boost your confidence by reminding yourself of past success—tests or projects that you aced. If you're putting as much effort into preparing for this test as you did for those, there's no reason you should expect to fail here. Work hard to prepare; then trust your preparation.

Second, surround yourself with encouraging people. It can be helpful to find a study group, but be sure that the people you're around will encourage a positive attitude. If you spend time with others who are anxious or cynical, this will only contribute to your own anxiety. Look for others who are motivated to study hard from a desire to succeed, not from a fear of failure.

Third, reward yourself. A test is physically and mentally tiring, even without anxiety, and it can be helpful to have something to look forward to. Plan an activity following the test, regardless of the outcome, such as going to a movie or getting ice cream.

When you are taking the test, if you find yourself beginning to feel anxious, remind yourself that you know the material. Visualize successfully completing the test. Then take a few deep, relaxing breaths and return to it. Work through the questions carefully but with confidence, knowing that you are capable of succeeding.

Developing a healthy mental approach to test taking will also aid in other areas of life. Test anxiety affects more than just the actual test—it can be damaging to your mental health and even contribute to depression. It's important to beat test anxiety before it becomes a problem for more than testing.

Study Strategy

Being prepared for the test is necessary to combat anxiety, but what does being prepared look like? You may study for hours on end and still not feel prepared. What you need is a strategy for test prep. The next few pages outline our recommended steps to help you plan out and conquer the challenge of preparation.

STEP 1: SCOPE OUT THE TEST

Learn everything you can about the format (multiple choice, essay, etc.) and what will be on the test. Gather any study materials, course outlines, or sample exams that may be available. Not only will this help you to prepare, but knowing what to expect can help to alleviate test anxiety.

STEP 2: MAP OUT THE MATERIAL

Look through the textbook or study guide and make note of how many chapters or sections it has. Then divide these over the time you have. For example, if a book has 15 chapters and you have five days to study, you need to cover three chapters each day. Even better, if you have the time, leave an extra day at the end for overall review after you have gone through the material in depth.

If time is limited, you may need to prioritize the material. Look through it and make note of which sections you think you already have a good grasp on, and which need review. While you are studying, skim quickly through the familiar sections and take more time on the challenging parts.

Write out your plan so you don't get lost as you go. Having a written plan also helps you feel more in control of the study, so anxiety is less likely to arise from feeling overwhelmed at the amount to cover.

STEP 3: GATHER YOUR TOOLS

Decide what study method works best for you. Do you prefer to highlight in the book as you study and then go back over the highlighted portions? Or do you type out notes of the important information? Or is it helpful to make flashcards that you can carry with you? Assemble the pens, index cards, highlighters, post-it notes, and any other materials you may need so you won't be distracted by getting up to find things while you study.

If you're having a hard time retaining the information or organizing your notes, experiment with different methods. For example, try color-coding by subject with colored pens, highlighters, or post-it notes. If you learn better by hearing, try recording yourself reading your notes so you can listen while in the car, working out, or simply sitting at your desk. Ask a friend to quiz you from your flashcards, or try teaching someone the material to solidify it in your mind.

STEP 4: CREATE YOUR ENVIRONMENT

It's important to avoid distractions while you study. This includes both the obvious distractions like visitors and the subtle distractions like an uncomfortable chair (or a too-comfortable couch that makes you want to fall asleep). Set up the best study environment possible: good lighting and a comfortable work area. If background music helps you focus, you may want to turn it on, but otherwise keep the room quiet. If you are using a computer to take notes, be sure you don't have any other windows open, especially applications like social media, games, or anything else that could distract you. Silence your phone and turn off notifications. Be sure to keep water close by so you stay hydrated while you study (but avoid unhealthy drinks and snacks).

Also, take into account the best time of day to study. Are you freshest first thing in the morning? Try to set aside some time then to work through the material. Is your mind clearer in the afternoon or evening? Schedule your study session then. Another method is to study at the same time of day that you will take the test, so that your brain gets used to working on the material at that time and will be ready to focus at test time.

STEP 5: STUDY!

Once you have done all the study preparation, it's time to settle into the actual studying. Sit down, take a few moments to settle your mind so you can focus, and begin to follow your study plan. Don't give in to distractions or let yourself procrastinate. This is your time to prepare so you'll be ready to fearlessly approach the test. Make the most of the time and stay focused.

Of course, you don't want to burn out. If you study too long you may find that you're not retaining the information very well. Take regular study breaks. For example, taking five minutes out of every hour to walk briskly, breathing deeply and swinging your arms, can help your mind stay fresh.

As you get to the end of each chapter or section, it's a good idea to do a quick review. Remind yourself of what you learned and work on any difficult parts. When you feel that you've mastered the material, move on to the next part. At the end of your study session, briefly skim through your notes again.

But while review is helpful, cramming last minute is NOT. If at all possible, work ahead so that you won't need to fit all your study into the last day. Cramming overloads your brain with more information than it can process and retain, and your tired mind may struggle to recall even previously learned information when it is overwhelmed with last-minute study. Also, the urgent nature of cramming and the stress placed on your brain contribute to anxiety. You'll be more likely to go to the test feeling unprepared and having trouble thinking clearly.

So don't cram, and don't stay up late before the test, even just to review your notes at a leisurely pace. Your brain needs rest more than it needs to go over the information again. In fact, plan to finish your studies by noon or early afternoon the day before the test. Give your brain the rest of the day to relax or focus on other things, and get a good night's sleep. Then you will be fresh for the test and better able to recall what you've studied.

STEP 6: TAKE A PRACTICE TEST

Many courses offer sample tests, either online or in the study materials. This is an excellent resource to check whether you have mastered the material, as well as to prepare for the test format and environment.

Check the test format ahead of time: the number of questions, the type (multiple choice, free response, etc.), and the time limit. Then create a plan for working through them. For example, if you have 30 minutes to take a 60-question test, your limit is 30 seconds per question. Spend less time on the questions you know well so that you can take more time on the difficult ones.

If you have time to take several practice tests, take the first one open book, with no time limit. Work through the questions at your own pace and make sure you fully understand them. Gradually work up to taking a test under test conditions: sit at a desk with all study materials put away and set a timer. Pace yourself to make sure you finish the test with time to spare and go back to check your answers if you have time.

After each test, check your answers. On the questions you missed, be sure you understand why you missed them. Did you misread the question (tests can use tricky wording)? Did you forget the information? Or was it something you hadn't learned? Go back and study any shaky areas that the practice tests reveal.

Taking these tests not only helps with your grade, but also aids in combating test anxiety. If you're already used to the test conditions, you're less likely to worry about it, and working through tests until you're scoring well gives you a confidence boost. Go through the practice tests until you feel comfortable, and then you can go into the test knowing that you're ready for it.

Test Tips

On test day, you should be confident, knowing that you've prepared well and are ready to answer the questions. But aside from preparation, there are several test day strategies you can employ to maximize your performance.

First, as stated before, get a good night's sleep the night before the test (and for several nights before that, if possible). Go into the test with a fresh, alert mind rather than staying up late to study.

Try not to change too much about your normal routine on the day of the test. It's important to eat a nutritious breakfast, but if you normally don't eat breakfast at all, consider eating just a protein bar. If you're a coffee drinker, go ahead and have your normal coffee. Just make sure you time it so that the caffeine doesn't wear off right in the middle of your test. Avoid sugary beverages, and drink enough water to stay hydrated but not so much that you need a restroom break 10 minutes into the test. If your test isn't first thing in the morning, consider going for a walk or doing a light workout before the test to get your blood flowing.

Allow yourself enough time to get ready, and leave for the test with plenty of time to spare so you won't have the anxiety of scrambling to arrive in time. Another reason to be early is to select a good seat. It's helpful to sit away from doors and windows, which can be distracting. Find a good seat, get out your supplies, and settle your mind before the test begins.

When the test begins, start by going over the instructions carefully, even if you already know what to expect. Make sure you avoid any careless mistakes by following the directions.

Then begin working through the questions, pacing yourself as you've practiced. If you're not sure on an answer, don't spend too much time on it, and don't let it shake your confidence. Either skip it and come back later, or eliminate as many wrong answers as possible and guess among the remaining ones. Don't dwell on these questions as you continue—put them out of your mind and focus on what lies ahead.

Be sure to read all of the answer choices, even if you're sure the first one is the right answer. Sometimes you'll find a better one if you keep reading. But don't second-guess yourself if you do immediately know the answer. Your gut instinct is usually right. Don't let test anxiety rob you of the information you know.

If you have time at the end of the test (and if the test format allows), go back and review your answers. Be cautious about changing any, since your first instinct tends to be correct, but make sure you didn't misread any of the questions or accidentally mark the wrong answer choice. Look over any you skipped and make an educated guess.

At the end, leave the test feeling confident. You've done your best, so don't waste time worrying about your performance or wishing you could change anything. Instead, celebrate the successful completion of this test. And finally, use this test to learn how to deal with anxiety even better next time.

> **Review Video: Test Anxiety**
> Visit mometrix.com/academy and enter code: 100340

Important Qualification

Not all anxiety is created equal. If your test anxiety is causing major issues in your life beyond the classroom or testing center, or if you are experiencing troubling physical symptoms related to your anxiety, it may be a sign of a serious physiological or psychological condition. If this sounds like your situation, we strongly encourage you to seek professional help.

Additional Bonus Material

Due to our efforts to try to keep this book to a manageable length, we've created a link that will give you access to all of your additional bonus material:

mometrix.com/bonus948/mblex

Made in the USA
Coppell, TX
11 July 2025

51625699R00138